CONQUEST

10 Simple Steps to Conquer Life and Leave a Lasting Legacy

AARON GENDLE

DOWNLOAD THE AUDIOBOOK FREE!

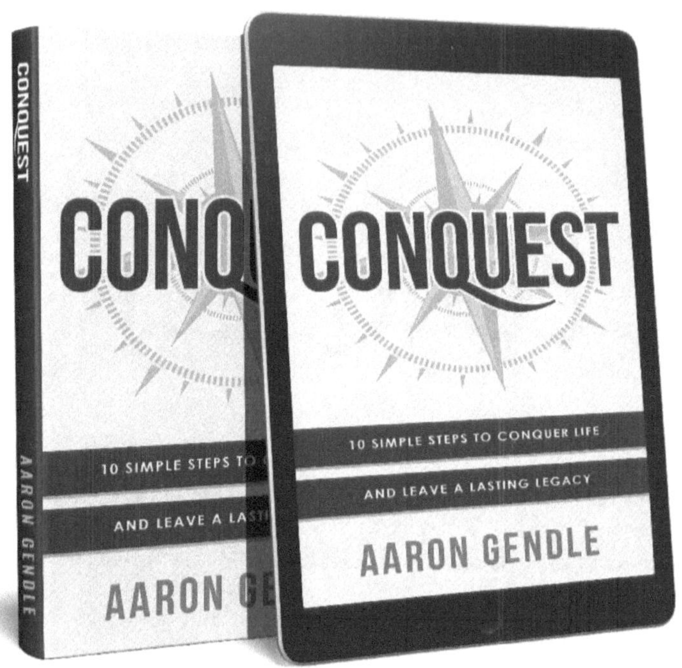

READ THIS FIRST

Just to say thanks for downloading my book, I would like to give you the Audiobook version 100% FREE!

Go to ...

https://writeabookuniversity.com/conquest-audiobook

WRITE A BOOK

UNIVERSITY

READY TO LEAVE YOUR LEGACY?

I believe one of the very best ways to leave your legacy and help others is to write a book.

No matter how young or old, it's never too soon or late to leave your mark on the world and

fulfill your dreams.

Get started writing your book today

with our FREE course.

Go to ...

https://writeabookuniversity.com/free

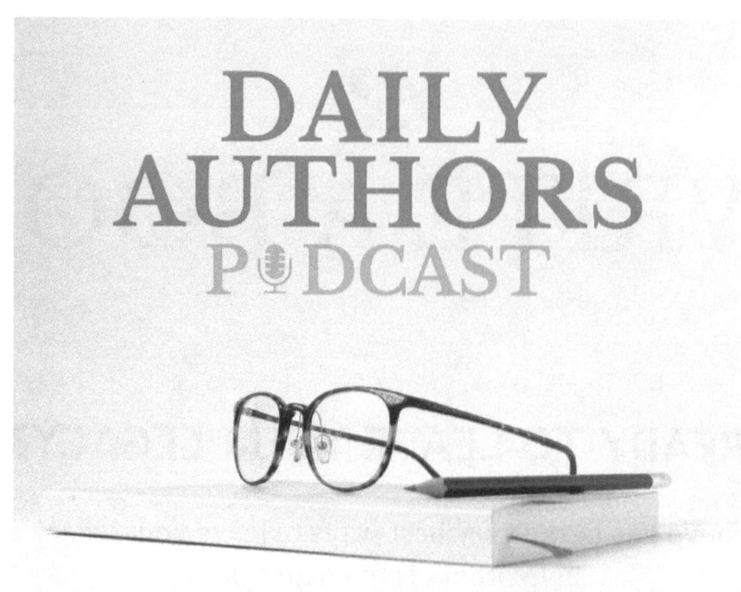

NEED SOME MORE INSPIRATION?

Listen to the **Daily Authors Podcast**. A daily podcast all about books and the authors who gave them life. Each episode, I interview a new, brilliant author, as they reveal inside information about their incredible books and inspiring lives.

Go to ...

dailyauthors.com

Dedications

My Amazing Wife Natalie

To my beautiful wife Natalie, for your support, encouragement, and love. Thanks for helping me think BIG. I love you so much.

My Kids

To my children, Violet, Oliver, Elliot, & Vivien. I wrote this thinking of you. I hope you'll read it one day and it will help you as much as it's helped me.

My Parents

To my parents, Tim and Belinda. I love you both.

Thanks for always believing in me.

Jason Tassi

In memory of Jason Tassi. I hope there is golf up in heaven and you are crushing it. You are missed and will always be remembered.

ISBN: 9781794071490

Aaron Gendle

Visit my websites

<u>Write a Book University</u>

writeabookuniversity.com

<u>Daily Authors Podcast</u>

dailyauthors.com

CONTENTS

CHAPTER 1

Introduction

"There is a winner in you. You were created to be successful, to accomplish your goals, to leave your mark on this generation. You have greatness in you. The key is to get it out."
– Joel Osteen

It was July, 2014. I was out for a run in the cornfields of Iowa with my lab mix, Roxy. After feeling the pressure of life that day, I needed to let off some steam.

My wife and two-year-old daughter had just moved cross country from Southern California to Ankeny, Iowa.

We just sold a condo we owned and were designing a custom home in Iowa, near my wife's family.

I was also starting a new job, and my son Oliver was about to be born. We had lots of amazing things happening in our life, but it was quite stressful at the same time.

On the final stretch of my run, I had an urge to use the restroom, #2 that is.

I got home just in time and did my business. Unfortunately, I had the green apple nasties, otherwise known as diarrhea.

I know, too much information. Sorry about that.

I didn't think much of it then, because I had spicy chicken wings the night before. However, the problem persisted and persisted. I also started getting bad stomach pain and cold sweats at night.

I'm not sure why it took me so long to go to the doctor, but about a month later, I figured I'd better go see what was wrong.

I was scared.

That's probably why it took me so long to go.

Gut Problems

Digging deeper, my suspicions led me to believe I had a serious, chronic, digestive disease called **Crohn's**.

Here's is how the Mayo Clinic describes Crohn's:

> *"It causes inflammation of your digestive tract, which can lead to abdominal pain, severe diarrhea, fatigue, weight loss and malnutrition. Inflammation caused by Crohn's disease can involve different areas of the digestive tract in different people.*
>
> *The inflammation caused by Crohn's disease often spreads deep into the layers of affected bowel tissue. Crohn's disease can be both painful and*

debilitating, and sometimes may lead to life-threatening complications."

After reading some of the online forum horror stories, I was terrified. Some treatments included the removal of parts of the intestine, or the entire colon and/or rectum.

Not cool.

Through some basic testing, my initial visit to urgent care only informed me of higher levels of inflammation in my body. So, it didn't reveal much, since the basic cold could have produced the same result.

I was told I needed a colonoscopy and would have to wait, in pain, until I could get one.

For those who don't know, a colonoscopy is where a camera is stuck up your butt to study your intestines. Yes, that's the technical definition.

Self-Reflection

While waiting to be tested, I began doing some hard thinking and self-reflection.

You see, just 6 months prior to my first symptoms, I was the owner of a surf inspired fitness gym in Huntington Beach, CA.

I was in the best shape of my life.

We sold the gym in expectation of moving back to Iowa.

While in great shape when I was running the gym, I stopped working out soon after selling the business and wasn't eating very well either. I also let moving, building a new home, starting a new job, and having a new baby, get to me.

I was stressed, big time!

Research Mode

From my initial research, I diagnosed myself with Crohn's disease, but was still waiting to get proper medical testing to confirm.

I dug through every forum, article, and google keyword search possible to find information on people who might have successfully battled Crohn's naturally.

You see, beyond having this disease, I was scared to death of the types of drugs I would be prescribed to put myself into remission.

Remission is simply a *state of lessening symptoms* or degree of symptoms.

The drugs most often used are immunosuppressants. They suppress your immune system, with the hope they suppress the parts of your immune system supposedly harming your intestines.

A major side effect being, bodily infections can become a huge ordeal. Not to mention all the other potential side effects and high drug costs.

I was highly motivated to heal myself naturally.

After some very late nights, I discovered some forum members talking about specific diets and how they used them to heal their bodies. I was then able to find doctors who had similar results with their clients.

While most physicians will state there isn't a real known cure for Crohn's medically, I had stumbled onto something that looked like, just that.

Success Strategy

My plan was simple, follow in the footsteps of people who had already won the battle with Crohn's, naturally.

> *"If you want to be successful, find someone who has achieved the results you want and copy what they do, and you'll achieve the same results."*
> —*Tony Robbins*

I won't go into all the details at this point in the book. I'll just say, a major part of the program was juicing. More on this in chapter 15.

When I started implementing the plan, I slowly began to feel better. My symptoms were diminishing.

Bad News

A month into this new lifestyle, I finally got a colonoscopy.

A week later, I got the call. A woman spoke in a calm voice and said, *"Aaron, you have Crohn's disease"*.

While I thought I had prepared myself mentally for that moment, it was surreal. I remember a rush of adrenaline and blood that put me into a haze.

To be told you have an incurable disease, sucks.

That day was a bit of a blur, but in the back of my mind, I had a plan, which gave me hope. I also had the support of my loving wife who was helping me with my new diet and lifestyle.

So, I kept at it.

Amazing Results

After a scheduling delay and an initial visit with a nurse a month or so after my colonoscopy, I finally met my gastroenterologist, or gut doctor, to discuss my disease.

He started by asking me, *"How do you feel?"*

I responded, *"I feel amazing. My symptoms are all gone."*

He seemed surprised. He responded with some additional questions to confirm and gave me some more background on the disease.

In about two or three minutes of talking he said, "Well, that's about all I know about Crohn's, but it looks like you're doing great. I've never had anyone come into my office after being diagnosed with Crohn's and tell me they no longer have symptoms. Whatever you are doing, keep it up!"

I was so relieved he was on my side and didn't try and push some drugs at me, seeing I was already symptom free.

He suggested I run the same inflammation test I took three months prior to confirm. So, I did, and the results came back successful. No signs of inflammation!

I felt like a million bucks and had far more energy and life than I did even before getting my first symptoms.

Here I am, over four years later, writing this book. Since then, I've been 99% symptom free, without any type of medication.

I would not claim I've found the cure for Crohn's, but damn close.

I recently competed in and successfully finished an Ultra Beast Spartan race. This race was 30 miles long with 60+ plus obstacles.

I feel so blessed to be healthy again! Not just to run obstacle races, but to have energy to play with my kids. To be there and provide for my family. To live life to the fullest.

Your Path to Success!

So, what does my success over Crohn's have to do with success in your life?

Great question!

First, let's clearly define success.

Webster describes it as A favorable or desired outcome; *also,* the attainment of wealth, favor, or eminence.

Therefore, success is simply obtaining a desired outcome.

Let me ask you, what is your desired outcome? What do you want out of life?

My desired outcome with Crohn's was to be free from its symptoms, if not cure it completely, through natural means alone.

I was dedicated, committed, and highly disciplined. I did whatever it took to accomplish my goal. I gave up all my unhealthy habits like fast food, drinking, coffee, bread, and the list goes on and on.

I sacrificed, big time, to succeed.

I don't say any of this to brag, but to simply demonstrate what is possible.

So, what are you willing to give up, to have success in your life?

Here is what I've discovered ...

My Crohn's success formula, what I now call, *Conquest*, has created success in many areas of my life.

So here is my hope for you reading this book.

If *Conquest* can conquer an incurable disease, I am confident it can help you succeed in your life.

The ten attributes of *Conquest* are:

1. Discovery
2. Passion & Desire
3. Belief
4. Goals
5. Fear, Doubt, & Action
6. Commitment
7. Research & Continual Learning
8. Health
9. Faith
10. Legacy

With these ten attributes, I've done and continue to do the impossible, and so can you.

These insights will help you conquer life by helping you believe in yourself, overcome your fears, discover your passion, upgrade your mind, transform your health, and leave a lasting legacy.

When these beliefs and habits become part of you, I'm certain the success you desire will become a reality.

Are you ready to begin your *Conquest*?

CHAPTER 2

Success is for Everyone

"All our dreams can come true if we have the
courage to pursue them."
– Walt Disney

I grew up fortunate enough to experience the wonderful world of Disneyland.

What a magical place and amazing rides:

- Haunted Mansion
- Splash Mountain
- Big Thunder Mountain Railroad
- Pirates of the Caribbean
- Peter Pan's Flight
- It's a Small World

I've ridden them all.

For about a year, my wife and I even had season passes. We loved taking my daughter Violet over to the park. We've had a blast at Disneyland.

I'm so glad Disney succeeded in building his dream park.

Walt Disney has an incredible story.

He received poor grades in school and even had to file for bankruptcy early in his career.

Disney was also rejected by over 300 banks when pitching his idea of Disneyland. We all know he persevered to build one of the most magical places on the planet.

Do you believe this type of success is possible for you?

Or, perhaps you've thought the success of others limits your opportunity.

Many of us don't believe success is within us and it's the same reason we aren't successful.

For a very long time, I thought my success was limited by the success of others. With Crohn's, I doubted whether the steps others took to succeed would work for me.

In other areas of my life, I also doubted whether I could be as successful as others.

I told myself, only limited amounts of success exists and huge success was too difficult or not even possible.

I would let negativity and regret take control, letting my thoughts limit my future.

Can you relate?

Do you have any of these doubts, yourself?

Do you ever think you're not worthy of the success you desire?

Do you sometimes make excuses that stop you in your tracks even before you attempt to succeed?

Now, I realize there are no limits to the success you and I can achieve.

We simply need the courage to dream and pursue those dreams.

Success is for everyone. Success is waiting for you.

Here are some success stories that should encourage you to believe prosperity is possible for you too.

Andrew Carnegie

Carnegie worked at a cotton mill for 12 hours a day, 6 days a week as a young boy.

After building his steel empire, he's now known as one of the wealthiest people ever and an incredible philanthropist.

Oprah Winfrey

Oprah, born into poverty, was a new mother at just 14 years old, after being molested at age 13. Her son died in infancy.

After dominating national television with *The Oprah Winfrey Show*, she grew her net worth to over 3 billion in 2017.

Sam Walton

Sam Walton grew up milking cows on the family farm in Oklahoma.

Later, Sam bought a Ben Franklin variety store, which eventually turned into the #1 retailer in the world, Walmart.

Joanne Rowling

Before creating the smashing success novel series, Harry Potter, JK Rowling suffered from clinical depression and was on welfare.

Rowling has now sold over 400 million copies of her books and has a net worth of around 1 billion dollars.

Jim Carrey

Jim Carrey didn't even finish high school and was living in his van when he started doing stand-up comedy routines.

Carrey eventually become one of the highest paid comedians in America.

Success is Waiting for You

Success is more than possible, it is yours for the taking. You don't need a PhD, money, or the right connections. You just need to believe and have the courage to pursue your dreams.

No matter who you are, where you are from, or how big your dream, success is waiting for you.

Just believe.

CHAPTER 3

Why You Must Succeed

"The world suffers a lot. Not because of the violence of bad people, but because of the silence of good people."
– Unknown

I sometimes wonder what my life would look like now had I decided to wait on doctors to tell me what was best for my health.

I am a member of many Crohn's related Facebook groups. I try and help support others who may want or need my help with their disease.

In these groups, I see many who are in deep depression. They have lost hope. They have given up.

On any given day, there's almost always someone looking for an alternative to the traditional prescribed drugs. You see, for many, these are just a Band-Aid. Drugs and surgeries have many side effects. Even if they do work, it can be short lived. The human body adapts, and their potency can wear off.

Others talk about how life is no longer worth living and curse the disease that has brought them so much pain. They have tried every medicine the doctors have thrown at them, removed major parts of their body, and are still in great pain.

The Painful Facts

Many of us are in great pain, with or without a chronic disease.

Are you in pain?

According to Time magazine, "Close to 13% of people 12 and older said they took an antidepressant in the last month."

As of 2017, an estimated 54% of people used illegal drugs in the previous 12 months.

In 2013, 30.2 percent of men and 16.0 percent of women, 12 and older, reported binge drinking in the past month.

According to the most recent data in 2017, adult obesity rates now exceed 35 percent in five states, 30 percent in 25 states, and 25 percent in 46 states.

There are close to 800,000 deaths due to suicide every year, which is one person every 40 seconds. Many more attempt suicide.

So, what does this mean?

This data tells me, the world is in pain. People are suffering and have lost hope.

Don't Give Up!

Are you suffering?

If you are, I encourage you with every fiber of my being, to keep going. Don't stop fighting. As Winston Churchill said, *"If you're going through hell, keep going"*

Why? Success is yours for the taking.

Moreover, the world needs you to succeed.

The world needs to hear your story. It needs your solutions. It needs your love. It needs all the amazing parts of you. It needs you to be your best.

Think of all the people that are hurting, you can help.

But if you don't succeed, your life will not nearly have the same impact. The great news is, you're reading this book now. You have taken that step.

When I first got sick, I would have loved to be handed the formula to conquer Crohn's.

Much in the same way, I am handing you the formula to succeed in life through my success, conquering an *"incurable"* disease.

I want you to understand, there's an incredible life waiting for you.

Don't give up, keep going, even if it feels like hell right now. Commit to more than average, and you'll experience the life you were meant for.

Become a Beacon of Hope

This new life offers so much more. In this life, you get to fulfill your dreams and positively affect the lives of everyone around you.

You'll be a beacon of hope for them and perhaps millions of others around the world.

So, you see, unless you succeed, you'll never get to experience life to its fullest or help others do the same.

You must succeed. The world is depending on you.

CHAPTER 4

Life is So Confusing

"Everybody gets so much information all day long that they
lose their common sense"
– Gertrude Stein

I grew up near the foothills in north central California. It was a quick hour or two car ride to some of the most beautiful places in the United States.

In just a few hours or less, I could be Monterey, San Francisco, Yosemite, and Napa, to name a few. If I wanted, I could surf and snowboard all in the same day.

Another memorable place was a small western style town called Jamestown. This is a former gold rush town where parts of Back to the Future 3, one of my all-time favorite movies, was filmed.

As a child, my parents would take us to Jamestown and meander around the quaint, old fashioned town. We would get an ice-cream cone and visit the candy shop. I loved visiting the gold mining store and gold troughs as well. We paid for a gold pan and would get to pan for gold like the old timers did.

I didn't realize this as a kid, but those old timers were sneaky. They would place a bit of gold in the troughs or pans with dirt they gave us, so we could find some gold in them.

It didn't matter, because it was a blast! I was so excited every time we went.

If you've ever panned for gold, then you know gold is heavier than most materials in the ground. So, to find it, you must shake the pan with some water, to allow the gold to sink to the bottom of the pan.

Then you swish the pan in the water to allow the lighter material to fall off the top layer.

You continue this process until you're left with the heaviest material and hopefully some gold at the bottom.

This childhood memory reminds me of the information age we live in.

So much information is created every single day. In fact, according to an IBM Marketing Cloud study, 90% of the data on the internet has been created in the last couple years. While this information can be a huge blessing, it can also be a curse.

Many of us are confused by so much data and rightly so. Who should we listen to? What information is accurate and what information is not?

We're distracted by buzzes, beeps, and alerts from our phones all day long. We take pictures, record videos, blog, post, like, share, upvote, tweet, and create so much information every second of the day.

Information is everywhere.

I've worked in the data consulting world for quite a while. My experience with data has shown me that many fortune 500 companies are also confused by their data.

Yes, they can move the data around and make it look pretty but figuring out what the data means is another thing. Comprehending data enough to make critical business decisions is very challenging, even for the best.

Are You Confused?

Are you confused by so much information?

If so, I completely understand. I was confused too.

When I started researching my cure to Crohn's, I felt very confused. There was so much conflicting information. Pharmaceutical companies stating their drug would do this and that or forums stating that proper nutrition and diet had little or nothing to do with the proper treatment of Crohn's.

I had to dig deep, then dig a little deeper. Through all the dirt, garbage, and mounds of information, at the bottom, were hidden nuggets of gold.

So, it's OK to be confused.

That's why I created this book.

I've spent dozens of hours sifting through a plethora of information to uncover hidden nuggets of gold. I did this, so you don't have to. So, I could hand you the keys to success.

Keep reading and I'll hand you those keys.

Ignite Your Imagination

"If you can dream it, you can do it."
– Walt Disney

Have you watched the movie *Field of Dreams,* with Kevin Costner?

This was one of my favorites growing up. Probably because it was about baseball, which I loved.

There's a famous quote from that movie where Costner is walking through his corn fields and hears a voice say, *"If you build it, he will come."*

The voice was urging Kevin's character Ray in the movie, to build a baseball field. So, he did.

When Ray built the baseball field, his wildest dreams came true. The ghosts of great baseball players began showing up playing baseball on his new baseball diamond.

Eventually, to his amazement, his father's ghost as a young man, also appeared. He was able to introduce his father's ghost to his family. Ray's wildest dreams had come true.

Why?

Because he believed it was possible and took action.

Now, Ray's dream is probably not your dream and I know this is just a fictional movie. However, after reading this book, internalizing the ten attributes of *Conquest*, and taking action, your dreams will come true too.

As young children, we have so much hope and so many dreams.

I started playing baseball at the age of four.

I grew up in the bay area in California and became an Oakland A's fan. I remember watching the bash brothers, Mark McGwire and Jose Canseco hit home runs. I watched Ricky Henderson steal bases and went to many major and minor league games.

Like so many young boys, I had big dreams of becoming a major league baseball player.

I asked my wife what she wanted to be as a child. She said, *"I wanted to be the first woman president!"*

What are your dreams?

Well, hopefully, you are still dreaming. But, many of us have stopped.

Why is it, as adults, we stop believing big things are possible?

Well, I believe it's because our mentors, parents, friends, and society tell us to be reasonable.

We're told not to get our hopes up or are influenced into living life like others who have given up on their dreams.

Then, we simply believe them. Why wouldn't we?

So, what can we do?

We need to rekindle the imagination we had as children.

Because, if we can't imagine, dream, or envision the success we want, unfortunately, it's not going to happen.

But, when we let ourselves dream and believe those dreams are possible, much like Walt Disney, our dreams will come true.

If possible, close your eyes right now and let your imagination run free. What is your biggest desire? What is your biggest dream?

Don't hold anything back.

This may be difficult to imagine. I know it has been for me. Our logical brain wants to immediately eliminate those crazy big dreams.

But don't let it!

You might tell yourself, "That's not possible, or maybe that can happen in 10 or 20 years down the road, but not now."

But, we didn't think that way as a child.

We imagined ourselves as baseball players or the first woman president, or whatever you dreamed of as a kid.

We didn't worry about whether it was realistic or not.

That's the same imagination we need as adults. So, continue to imagine your wildest dreams and let go of any doubt.

Our minds are built to see images. Build those images of yourself already accomplishing your wildest dreams.

That is what I want for you and what you'll be able to make a reality after applying *Conquest* to your life.

The Big Picture

"If you just focus on the smallest details,
you never get the big picture right."
– Leroy Hood

There are ten elements of *Conquest*. I have positioned these attributes in order of how I experienced them fighting Crohn's. This is a similar order you might also experience *Conquest* in your life.

But before we dive deeper into *Conquest*, let's take a quick high-level look at each success element.

Step 1 - Discovery

Discovery is a very important part of *Conquest*.

Discovery is about self-reflection. We must take a deep look within ourselves to understand what's not working and what life we truly want.

Once we acknowledge something needs to change, like I did with Crohn's, we're able to address our shortcomings and discover our true desires.

Do not skip this critical first step to success.

Find out more about discovery in Chapter 8.

Step 2 - Passion and Desire

Finding your passion is easier than you might think. The difficult part is overcoming the urge to deny our obsessions.

As children we have big dreams, but as adults we tend to suffocate our dreams.

By digging deep within and asking yourself some critical questions, you'll uncover your desires.

I'll help you with these questions in Chapter 9.

Step 3 - Believe

Our thoughts create our reality. You have probably heard of the placebo effect.

This is where positive or negative symptoms occur in an individual who has taken a placebo pill or shot.

A placebo does not contain any active ingredients that could help or hurt a person. So how do individuals receive positive or negative symptoms?

Through the mind.

The mind creates expectations that can alter body chemistry.

We believe we're getting better, so we get better. Conversely, we might believe we're getting sicker, so we do.

Don't underestimate the power of belief.

You can read more about the power of belief in chapter 10.

Step 4 - Big & Scary Goals

What are your goals?

Do you have any?

A Harvard study suggests 83% of the US population do not have goals.

How can we achieve success if we have not defined what that means to us?

Moreover, according to a study by Dr. Gail Matthies, we're 42% more likely to achieve our goals when we write them down.

Beyond a lack of goal setting and writing them down, many goals tend to be tiny. Small goals do not inspire us to achieve them.

So, how do we fix this problem?

We'll get into the nitty gritty in chapter 11.

Step 5 - Fear, Doubt, & Action

What fear, and doubts are keeping you from the success you desire?

I've heard it said, that thing we most fear is what we most need to do. In my experience, this has been a soberingly, accurate statement.

Action is the key to overcoming our fear and doubt.

We'll discuss fear, doubt, and action more in chapter 12.

Step 6 - Commit

Have you committed to the success you desire?

If so, great, you are well on your way to succeeding. If not, what's holding you back?

Have you found the deeper purpose behind your goals? Have you found your why?

Without 100% commitment daily, you're likely to fall short of your desired outcome.

Don't just hope, commit and make it happen. More about committing in chapter 13.

Step 7 - Research & Continual Learning

Congrats on reaching this far into the book. You are obviously one that takes learning seriously and I commend you for that.

Research and continual learning have been essential to my *Conquest* over Crohn's as well as many other successes in my life.

We'll take a deeper dive into this element in chapter 14, but I want you to know this drive for knowledge will propel you further than you can imagine.

So, keep reading and learning.

Step 8 - Health

Without my health I wouldn't be writing these words right now.

I believe deeply in each element of *Conquest*, but I might have to say that health is one of the greatest contributors to success.

It's essential.

Without our health, we don't have much.

Within chapter 15, I'll be revealing my health tips and secrets to overcoming an incurable disease. My hope is you'll be able to leverage this information and use it to better your health, no matter how good or bad it is.

Step 9 - Faith

Do you believe in something bigger than yourself?

Where do you turn when life is too much to handle?

Without a greater purpose and bigger meaning, life can be empty and overwhelming.

When the burden of life is so great, faith can help you be victorious.

When your dreams are so close you can taste them, faith will take you all the way.

If you would like to discover a deeper purpose for your life or see how faith can get you closer to your dreams, make sure to read chapter 16.

Step 10 - Legacy

After going into complete remission and gaining huge success with my health, I realize I have something massive to offer the world.

Beyond the specific steps I took to heal myself, I'm very excited to share my journey to success with you now.

I'm excited for my young kids to grow up and read this book, years from now.

I know these words will be around long after I am not, helping others live a big life.

I also have plans to write dozens more books to help and inspire thousands, if not millions, of people around the world.

While this phase can begin at any point during your journey, the last element of success is legacy.

Have you ever asked yourself, "If I die tomorrow, what will my legacy be?"

"What will others remember me for?"

"Will I be remembered at all?"

You see, sharing our success with others is what makes us successful. Helping others do what we have been able to accomplish is an essential part of success.

This element of *Conquest* will help you unlock your legacy and ensure you live on to help others, forever.

One of the very best ways I believe you can leave your legacy is by writing a book.

For this reason, I've started <u>writeabookuniversity.com</u>. So, if you choose, you can leave your legacy by writing a book and I'll be there to help you do just that.

Pro Step - Remember Like a Ninja

I know I mentioned there were just 10 steps to *Conquest*, but I wanted to give you just one more, memory.

We are what we remember. The sad part is, we tend to forget quite a bit.

Well, in chapter 17, I'll show you some ninja memory tricks that helped me ace college tests, remember names on demand, and anything else I wanted to remember.

I'll also give you an easy way to remember the ten elements of *Conquest*. Use these tricks to remember your favorite books, lists, names, and much more.

CHAPTER 7

It's Time to Prepare

"Before anything else, preparation is the key to success."
– Alexander Graham Bell

It had been a long road, but we finally made it. High school soccer section finals were here.

Our rivals, Ripon Christian Academy, a strong all Dutch team from a neighboring city.

Earlier the same year, this team crushed us with a double-digit win.

If you aren't familiar with the game of soccer, reaching double digits is quite ridiculous.

But, our team had made major improvements over the season and somehow made it to the finals.

This was it. One game for all the glory and bragging rights. The season championship.

Our opponents were big and tall. The goalie was 6 feet 5 inches, at least.

They were intimidating and challenging to score on.

The whistle blew, and the championship began.

Later in the game, it started to sprinkle. I knew this would make any shots more difficult to stop, since the ball would be wet and slippery.

I was passed the ball, but quite a long way from the goal. Not a typical distance I would take a shot from.

However, at that moment, something my coach always preached buzzed through my mind.

Not the words of my high school soccer coach, but my club soccer coach.

You see, I had been playing soccer since I was 4 years old.

At this time in my soccer career, I played soccer year-round on one of the very best soccer teams in California.

We were State Champions for several years, trained several times a week, and would play upwards of 80 games a year.

So what words did I remember?

My coach always told us to challenge the goalie no matter what. To make him stop the ball by putting a shot on goal. A shot that if he didn't stop, would score. Even if the shot wasn't the most powerful, it would never do any good if it wasn't on goal.

So, I took the long shot. I kept my head down through the strike, but after the ball was away, I looked up. It was a solid strike. The ball was driven low to the ground and just barely skipped by the diving goalie's fingertips, landing perfectly in the left side of the net.

It was an amazing moment. I went on to score two goals that game as we won three goals to zero.

So, was it all a fluke? How did we beat a team that earlier the same year destroyed us? How did I score two goals that game?

Yes, you guessed it, preparation.

During our soccer season, our team became a lot tighter. Our skills were more developed. The hours of practice and playing prepared us to win the championship.

The same is true in life and in this book. I want to prepare you for the upcoming sections and chapters. I want to prepare you to succeed in life.

In college, I did quite a bit of weight lifting.

We've probably all heard the saying, *"No pain, no gain"*, when it comes to working out.

This saying always made sense to me from a physical standpoint. However, over time, I've realized, mental and emotional challenges are also good for us.

Your personal path to *Conquest* will challenge you mentally, emotionally, and physically.

Mental and Emotional Prep

We have done some mental and emotional preparation already, but let's make sure we're on the same page.

One of the biggest problems I had when I began my journey of personal growth and success, was skepticism.

It was easy for me to feel like I was already on the path to success. This is a dangerous place to be.

When I was diagnosed, I had what many would consider success, married to my beautiful wife Natalie with two amazing children.

We owned a beautiful white picket home. I had a great career that brought in a solid income.

But, one of my biggest regrets in life is acting like I had things figured out.

There was a long period of my life where I stopped growing as a person. Sure, I enhanced many of the skills necessary to advance my career, but I had given up on self-development.

I was blessed enough to have an amazing wife who was constantly listening to and reading book after book.

She kept insisting I read this book or listen to that podcast. I always told her I would, and many times I would do so partially, but my heart was never in it.

I was a skeptic.

However, very slowly, she kept chipping away at me until I began to realize how little I knew.

Observe the quote by Donald Rumsfeld:

> *"There are known knowns. These are things we know that we know. There are known unknowns. That is to say, there are things that we know we don't know. But there are also unknown*

I think we can all agree, we don't know what we don't know.

So, don't be a skeptic like I was.

Don't let the success you've already achieved in life keep you from achieving even greater success.

Open your mind to the possibility that you don't know something. That small gap will clear the way for new information and ideas that weren't there before.

It just takes one great idea to change the course of your life forever.

Physical Prep

One of the ten elements of *Conquest* I'll be discussing is health.

This book is about my journey in overcoming some major health issues, so that makes sense, right?

No, I'm not going to ask you to do 100 pushups or anything like that.

Believe it or not, I did very minimal exercise to regain my physical health on my journey to conquer Crohn's.

Most importantly, it was what I put in my body and how I managed stress.

The advice I'll be sharing will be a challenge. So, I want you to mentally prepare yourself for the physical challenges ahead.

Yes, success is waiting for you, but it comes at a cost.

Is the cost worth it?

Yes, I've no doubt it is well worth it.

The choices for me with Crohn's were:

1. Continue my unhealthy habits and hope that some expensive pill or shot will help me feel a little better. Most likely, I would have to learn to just live with the pain of Crohn's.
2. Do a 180 with my lifestyle and have a chance of never needing to take medication and feel better than I did before getting sick.

I obviously chose option #2 and have not looked back since.

Open Your Heart

Do you have health problems?

Well, I hope you're already on a path to fantastic health, but for many this is not the case.

The #1 killer, heart disease, is almost entirely treatable by lifestyle changes alone.

The answer is so simple.

Then why are so many dying of it you might ask?

I been asked this same question about Crohn's in Facebook forums after explaining my simple self-healing recipe (see chapter 15 for more details).

From hours spent researching and chatting to others with Crohn's, here is what I discovered:

1. We don't know the solution.

2. We received bad information and are following the wrong solution.
3. We have the right solution, but are skeptical or doubt it will work, so we never take action.
4. We have the right solution, but are unwilling to make the sacrifices necessary to succeed.
5. We have the right solution and are taking the necessary action to succeed.

So what group are you in?

Since you're reading this book, you'll have to eliminate #1 and #2. You won't be able to claim ignorance and you will have the right solution.

But, will you be a skeptic? Are you willing to make the sacrifices necessary to succeed?

Prepare your heart, mind, and soul for success.

Open your heart to the possibility of learning something life changing in this book. Prepare your mind for the mental and physical challenges necessary to succeed. Once you understand what you need to do, commit 100% and you will succeed.

CHAPTER 8

Discovery

(STEP 1)

"Without reflection, we go blindly on our way,
creating more unintended consequences, and
failing to achieve anything useful."
– Margaret J. Wheatley

I've worked in the IT and consulting world for over twelve years.

One of the very first steps I always take to find out how I can help a customer is discovery.

With each new project, I sat down with business and technology personnel to understand their problems and help them design a solution.

This portion of the project was always critical.

Without proper requirements and design, we could very easily spend hundreds of hours and millions of dollars building something the customer does not want.

Many companies have now adopted what's called an agile development methodology.

This means the group in charge of designing and creating the solution works alongside its customers in short time intervals. They demonstrate to the business their progress on a regular basis, every two weeks, generally.

The main reason for this is to get feedback quickly and ensure the right solution is being created. If there's a problem, it's much easier to correct two weeks' worth of work, than two months' worth of work.

If discovery works for some of the most successful companies in the world, shouldn't this work for our own lives?

Many of us go through life without much self-reflection or discovery. We don't realize how bad our situation is. We ignore the obvious signs and symptoms that something isn't right.

We are so used to living out our daily routines, we trick ourselves into believing life is ok. I'm not saying we envision our life is a fairy tale, but we fool ourselves into believing the mundane or average are fine.

This results in a lack of urgency to make changes.

What Symptoms Are You Experiencing?

With Crohn's, I first discovered something was wrong after my jog that summer evening.

While having obvious physical symptoms made my problem easier to identify and created urgency, you most likely have symptoms of your own.

You may not have a chronic disease, but you may not be happy with your career, family life, financial situation, or physical health.

Unless we hit rock bottom, it's easy to simply tolerate our lives.

Almost all problems have symptoms. These potential symptoms may include: depression, emptiness, loneliness, anger, frustration, weight gain, stress, physical ailments, and difficulty sleeping.

So, the first step to success is self-reflection and discovery.

I love this quote by Alan Cohen:

> *"Everyone and everything that shows up in our life is a reflection of something that is happening inside of us."*

We must first acknowledge something's not right. That something needs to change.

If I had kept ignoring my body screaming it wasn't happy, I would never have started the journey to heal myself. Quite the opposite. I am certain I would have gotten sicker and sicker.

Stop Blaming Others

Another area I've seen this in my life is with my marriage.

I've been married for almost 12 years now and yes, there have been ups and downs.

We have had some amazing moments, but there have also been many arguments and disagreements, even threats of divorce.

These were some obvious symptoms of major problems.

The tendency I have observed in myself and others, is, we don't like to blame ourselves.

Sure, there may be some obvious challenges with your partner or spouse, but have you acknowledged your own problems.

I spent many years only looking at my wife's problems and not my own. This always caused resentment, anger, and frustration.

You see, the successful do not blame others for their problems. They take responsibility for everything in their life, good and bad.

I could have blamed my genetics or food companies for my disease.

Even if these contributed to some degree, it wouldn't do me any good to cast blame. It would not make me feel better or heal my gut to do so.

Instead, I took the blame and responsibility for my problems.

With my marriage, I thought about whether I was making my wife feel important. How could I make her feel important every day? What areas in my life could I improve to connect more with her? What could I do to have an amazing marriage?

With my disease, I asked myself, what am I eating? What am I doing to manage my stress? Am I living a healthy lifestyle? What can I do to heal myself and feel even better than I did before getting sick?

This self-reflection and discovery have saved my marriage and health.

Reflect on Your Life

So, what symptoms do you have?

Are you living the life you want?

Take time right now to reflect on your life. Make this a daily habit. Go on a long walk at night or find some quiet time before rushing into your busy day.

This is important.

Don't worry about fixing any problems at this point.

Simply ask yourself, what are the signs and symptoms of my life? Is there something I need to address or change?

Are you angry, depressed, lonely, or broke?

Acknowledge your life isn't what you want it to be and why. Then ask, what have I done to create these symptoms?

What excuses have I created that prevent me from being successful?

This will be the challenging part. Like I said before, it goes against human nature to see our own problems, but you must take responsibility.

Don't blame anyone else. Get rid of all excuses.

I encourage you to spend whatever time you need asking yourself these questions before moving onto the next chapter.

Once you've discovered the areas that need improvement and taken responsibility for your life, you'll be able to find solutions and create the life you desire.

Your heart and mind will be open to change.

You'll be open to finding your true desires and discovering the exciting life you're after.

Here are your key takeaways:

- The successful self-reflect and never blame others.
- Ask yourself, what are the symptoms of my life?
- By reflecting on our lives, we can address any issues holding us back from real success.

CHAPTER 9

Find Your Passion & Fuel Your Desires

(STEP 2)

"You know you are on the road to success if you would do your job, and not be paid for it."
– Oprah Winfrey

When I was a kid, I had a couple of big passions, playing the piano and golf.

I devoted hundreds of hours to both activities and loved every minute of it.

It never crossed my mind to get paid for any of these activities. Sure, I played some gigs here and there that made a few bucks or got a free meal, but it was never the incentive.

Then, I grew up and society told me I needed to make money, and should go to college to get a job that pays the bills.

So, I did. Now what?

Many of us wake up in the middle of our careers lacking purpose. Our jobs become a means to an end. We punch the clock and work for the weekends.

Sound familiar?

Well, after we've done some discovery and self-reflection, we need to better understand our desires.

We've acknowledged something's not right, but what do we do next?

With Crohn's, my desire was clear, rid myself of the disease and/or its symptoms, naturally.

I was hyper-motivated. I spent hundreds of hours, almost all my extra time, trying to figure out how to heal myself. I was very passionate.

Unless you have a chronic disease, your desires may not be so obvious. For example, you might discover you no longer like your job or career path. But, it's not always so evident what your career path should be.

That's why discovering your passion is so important.

What You Are Excited About Right Now?

I've tried to make money in lots of ways. But I've always been the most satisfied doing what I enjoyed.

For a short period of time, my family and I were renting out our home on popular rental websites like Airbnb and HomeAway.

We were making great extra money. We had two properties and would jump back and forth between our main residence and other rental property depending on which one was booked.

It was very profitable. However, it put a huge strain on our family. We were moving back and forth all while maintaining our careers and two young children.

We had to get the properties cleaned and be prepared to spend three days to a week at one of our residence's multiple times a month.

This was a huge lesson for me. While the money was great, in the end, it was not worth it. Now, I'm not saying that you should be happy simply working a 9 to 5 job you don't like for a boss you despise.

No, quite the opposite. Both situations are similar. If you aren't doing something that excites you, or something you're passionate about, then it's probably time to move on.

Let me be clear however, this doesn't mean you have to figure out your life-long calling today. Life is a journey. One step takes us to the next.

Try to focus on what you're most excited about right now.

When I first began my journey to conquer Crohn's, it was all I could think about. I was overwhelmed with the excitement and possibility of conquering this disease. Now I am writing a book about how I defeated Crohn's and the success secrets I discovered along the way.

However, when I began trying to find a way to heal myself, I wasn't thinking about writing a book to help others conquer Crohn's and life.

The process of healing myself, staying healthy, and growing as an individual has allowed me to share this information with you today.

Find Your Passion

So, how do you find your passion?

Well, I love what Grant Cardone says in a Forbes interview about his book, *Be Obsessed or Be Average:*

> *"Find something, anything, that you're obsessed with and quit denying it. Own it and feed it because it has massive amounts of energy and creativity. Make a list of all the greats that have walked this planet and you will see they simply embraced their obsessions. They didn't apologize or try to make others comfortable, they embraced their obsessions and poured everything into them."*

To find your passion, ask yourself these questions:

"What are you obsessed over?"

"What obsessions have you denied in your life?"

"What do you do now for free, simply because you love it?"

"What were you passionate about as a child?"

"What excites you right now?"

"What do you want people to know you for?"

"What are you good at?"

"What do other people say you're good at?"

Spend some time asking yourself these questions and I am certain you'll begin to uncover your passions and path to success.

Here are your key takeaways:

- Life is a journey. Let your passions guide you. Understand where you want to go by understanding what you're passionate about.
- To find your passion, start by ask yourself the list of questions mentioned in this chapter.
- Embrace your passions and do not deny them.

Just Believe

(STEP 3)

"Man often becomes what he believes himself to be. If I keep on saying to myself that I cannot do a certain thing, it is possible that I may end by really becoming incapable of doing it. On the contrary, if I shall have the belief that I can do it, I shall surely acquire the capacity to do it, even if I may not have it at the beginning."
– Mahatma Gandhi

It was a Monday night and the tournament was on. I was ready to show off my skills. My team partner and I were excited to win it all. It was cornhole time.

What is cornhole you might ask?

Well, here is the official definition from Wikipedia:

"Cornhole (also known as dummy boards, bean bag toss, dadhole, doghouse, Baggo, Arse-bag,

Sack Toss, or corn hole) is a lawn game in which players take turns throwing bags of corn (or bean bags) at a raised platform with a hole in the far end. A bag in the hole scores 3 points, while one on the platform scores 1 point. Play continues until a team or player reaches (or exceeds) the score of 21."

This game is very popular in Iowa, where I used to live. In fact, the game was invented in the Midwest.

I had found a local meetup group that was putting on a charity tournament at a downtown brewery.

I texted my brother-in-law a few days prior to see if he wanted to partner up. He was in. Game on.

At last, it was Monday night and we were ready to go. The first game began.

My first four bag tosses were OK at best. I hit the board with two of them, but our opponents were on fire. My turn came up again and tossed my next four bags. Not one of them stuck on the board.

Ouch!

My partner kept us in the match for one more round.

It was my turn once again. Our opponent scored the necessary points to win, but I could keep us in the match by landing one or more bags on the board.

So, what happened next? I missed the board four more times in a row.

Chalk up loss number one.

Luckily, it was a double elimination tournament. So, I had a chance to redeem myself.

It was ten minutes or so before it was our turn once again. In those ten minutes I did some thinking. I also had a beer to calm my nerves a bit.

I started to imagine some of the past bags games I had won. I envisioned the bag going in the hole and imagined having perfect technique. I could feel my confidence come back. Then, I just believed we could win.

The next game was a night and day difference. I began to land almost every bag either on the board or in the hole. Some rounds, I was able to get three bags in the hole in a row.

While we didn't win the tournament, we won our next two games and should have won our third.

However, this story isn't about winning, it's about believing.

What was the difference between the first game and the ones thereafter?

Yes, you guessed it, *belief.*

When I began to believe, it became my reality. With each bag that landed on the board or went in the hole, I believed some more.

With each win, I believed we could win some more.

The same belief held true during my fight with Crohn's. But, I didn't believe right away. I was very discouraged, doubtful, and depressed.

It took time. Eventually, I allowed myself to believe I could be healed naturally.

That belief gave me hope and motivation to keep at it.

Belief inspired me to continue searching for the right solution. With each incremental improvement in my health, my belief became stronger.

By believing I could conquer the incurable, I did just that.

Surf's Up

For my 30th birthday, we decided to get out of Iowa, and head off to southern California where I spent some of my college years. I had many friends there and knew it would be a blast to hang out with them all.

My parents also came down from northern California and stayed in their camper at a local RV Park. The park had a great location, right across the street from some of the best surfing in United States.

We were staying at a nearby hotel but would visit my parent in their camper at the park on occasion.

One evening, my wife and I went to the RV Park's public spa to relax. We met a couple jolly characters who were also relaxing in the spa. We struck up a conversation and discovered these guys lived at the park. For a relatively low rate, they were able to live their dream beach life.

Soon, the trip was over. We had a great visit and headed back to Iowa. On our flight back, my wife and I started chatting.

Every time we travel, we got inspired to do big things. This time, my wife said, *"why don't we get a camper, and go live on the beach?"*

At first, I was skeptical and didn't know if she was even serious. But, after some more chatting, the idea started growing on me. I missed surfing, the wonderful weather, and the beautiful beaches.

So, we decided to go for it.

We didn't know how we would do it. We knew we had many hurdles and roadblocks that could get in our way, but we were going try our best to make it happen.

Airstream

First, we needed a camper!

We looked and looked. My wife and I were fond of Airstreams, but many were out of our budget. We eventually found an old 60s airstream in decent shape, but it was all the way down in Mississippi. Mississippi was about thirteen hours away from us.

I spoke to my brother-in-law Kyle to see if he was up for an adventure. I knew it would be tough to take that journey up and back to Iowa by myself. He was game, so we set off to get our camper.

We did the drive up and back in less than 30 hours. We drove non-stop all the way there, took a half hour nap on the beach, got the camper, then drove right back up to Iowa.

The camper was in decent shape on the outside, but it needed lots of work on the inside. Still not knowing if we would make it to the beach, we spent the summer fixing it up in preparation.

Our Home

Next, we had to figure out what to do with our beautiful home in Iowa. We didn't want to sell it, so we decided to rent it out.

We worked out a deal with my brother-in-law to rent and take care of our home. Another task off the list.

I Need a v8

Another big to do was our vehicle. I had a Toyota Tacoma at the time, but it just wasn't big enough to tow our Airstream cross country. So, I needed to sell it and buy a new truck. Easy right?

Well, turns out it was. I put my Tacoma on Craigslist, and sold it in about a week. Then, I found a used Ford 150 with a v8. Done and done.

Money

Now the last big hurdle was my job. You see, I had a decent paying gig in Iowa as a data guy. I had done a good job for the company and thought, instead of finding a new job, why don't I simply ask to work remotely.

I worked up some courage and just weeks before we were planning on leaving, I convinced my employer to let me keep my job and work remotely.

We Did It!

I remember calling my wife after that conversation at work and being so excited. *"We did it"*, we said to one another. We were going to live by the beach.

We drove cross country just weeks later, less than 4 months from that initial trip to southern California.

So, how did we do it?

Yes, you guessed it, we believed.

Sure, we had some doubts along the way, but as each obstacle was overcome, our doubts diminished. Each time we checked a to do off our list, we knew we were one step closer to our dream.

We had a blast living by the beach. We even started the surf inspired fitness gym I mentioned in the introduction. We made our dreams a reality because we believed it was possible.

Do You Believe?

So, do you believe, or have you stopped believing?

Maybe life has tossed you around a bit and your not where you thought you would be. Let me encourage you to forget about past and look to the future.

Your dreams are waiting for you to reach out and grab them, but first, you must believe.

Say these words out loud with me right now:

"I believe."

"All of my dreams are coming true."

"This is the best day of my life."

"I am blessed."

"Nothing can stop me from achieving my dreams."

"Success is headed my way."

I love this quote by David Schwartz:

> *"Believe it can be done. When you believe something can be done, really believe, your mind will find the ways to do it. Believing a solution paves the way to solution."*

I hope it inspires you to believe all your dreams are possible.

Here are your key takeaways:

- Your mind is a powerful tool.
- To succeed, you must first believe it is possible.
- Disbelief will keep you from succeeding.
- Remind yourself out lout that all your dreams are coming true.

CHAPTER 11

Set Big & Scary Goals

(STEP 4)

"People are not lazy. They simply have impotent goals - that is, goals that do not inspire them."
– Tony Robbins

It's almost that time of year again, New Year's. At the time of writing this book, the new year is less than 1 month away.

It's the time of year many goals are set.

Unfortunately, most of these goals are never accomplished.

A study from the University of Scranton suggests that only 8% of us will achieve our resolution goals.

Why?

Well, I believe a major reason is because our new year's goals are not big and exciting enough.

Let's look at another quote by Grant Cardone:

"The single biggest financial mistake I've made was not thinking big enough. I encourage you to go for more than a million. There's no shortage of money on this planet, only a shortage of people thinking big enough."

The answer is simple, think big and set massive goals, goals that excite you. Big goals are going to excite you into action, not little dinky goals.

Burst of Energy

I love running with my dog Roxy.

Towards the end of our run, Roxy and I will both be tired.

Naturally, right?

But, I noticed something the other day I found quite interesting. As we're wrapping up our run, occasionally we'll see a cat, rabbit, squirrel, or another dog.

When that happens, Roxy will get a burst of energy and attempt to catch the animal she sees. I hold her back of course, but it's amazing how much energy she has. It's as if we had just started the run.

The point being, she sees something that excites her, and it propels her forward regardless of being exhausted seconds before.

As humans, I believe we're the same way. We get tired. Some days are too long. We just want to sit down on the couch and relax, right?

Well, there's nothing wrong with relaxing. But, if we find that thing that excites us, we're going to have the energy to accelerate towards it. We'll have endless energy and motivation to accomplish our goals and achieve our dreams.

When I was sick, I had a massive goal to conquer the incurable.

The thought of being healthy again or even healthier than I was before getting sick, was very exciting.

I could have set some smaller goals like:

- Learn to live with my disease and mentally accept my new condition.
- Or, get into remission through drugs after several months.

I didn't set any of these goals because they were just too small.

The results were not exciting. I wanted to live life like this disease had never been part of me. So, I set a goal to eliminate all symptoms, without any medication, as fast as I could, naturally.

At the time, I didn't know how long it would take. It turns out, it only took a few months!

Do Your Goals Scare You?

There's another key to a successful goal, a goal that scares you.

Here is another quote I love by Joe Vitale:

> *"A goal should scare you a little and excite you a lot."*

I like to think about this quote in a couple different ways:

1. Something that takes you out of your comfort zone.
2. Goals that scare you if you don't accomplish them.

Out of Your Comfort Zone

Goals should be scary enough to take us out of our comfort zone. They should try and push us to another level in life. They need to be big enough to scare us.

For example, I recently set and accomplished a big goal to run an Ultra Beast Spartan race. It's 30 miles with 60+ obstacles. For a while, I was simply going to sign up for a shorter race. There isn't anything wrong with doing those of course. They are all tough.

However, none of the other shorter races scared me. So, that's how I knew I needed to sign up and defeat the Ultra Beast.

Too Scared to Stop

Goals should also scare you to never stop.

When I was sick, I was very scared. I was scared I wouldn't be able to play with my kids. I was scared I wouldn't be able to provide for my family. I feared being a burden. I was afraid of how sick I might get.

So, I set a huge goal to conquer Crohn's. Yes, this goal alone was scary, but I was also scared of what would happen if I didn't succeed.

The same is true when I set off to write this book. I thought to myself, *"what will happen if I don't write?"*

I thought of my kids. Maybe this book would help prevent them from making the same mistakes and getting a disease like this. Or, it could help them overcome other challenges in their lives.

I thought of others with Crohn's, ones that I had been chatting with on Facebook groups. The one's looking for solutions that needed more than an instant message of encouragement or brief advise. I thought, *"how many of them would suffer their entire lives if I didn't share my story?"*

Lastly, I thought of all the others who would be encouraged to do big things, and go for their dreams. How many of them would fall short of their dreams if I did not write this book? That meant they wouldn't be able to help even more people.

So, set scary goals, the world is depending on you!

A Big Purpose

Another lesson I learned about goals is that big goals should also have a big purpose.

Yes, I was motivated to heal myself for my own quality of life, but I had an even greater motivation.

I needed to provide for my young family. I wanted to have the energy to play with my daughter and newborn son. I wanted to be there for them and I didn't want some crappy disease sucking the life from me.

With every big goal I've set and accomplished, there has always been a bigger purpose that's driven me to succeed.

With each goal you write, I challenge you to ask yourself why you want to accomplish that goal.

Then, whatever you answer, ask yourself why again.

Ask yourself why seven times, and you'll have your deeper purpose for each goal. This is an awesome exercise I've learned from reading *Millionaire Success Habits*, by Dean Graziosi.

This exercise is best done with a partner.

Our first answer to this "Why" question is likely to be only a surface level reason. We need to continue asking ourselves why to get down to the real answer.

Once we have that why, let it remind you every time you lack motivation or inspiration. Let that why be the reason you wake up each morning.

I Am …

Writing your goals down is critical.

Did you know that people with written goals are 42% more likely to achieve their goals?

Incredibly, just 14% of people have a goal plan in mind, but never write them down.

Only 3 out of every 100 adults write their goals down on paper.

Moreover, sharing your goals with a close friend or someone to hold you accountable is proven to increase the chances of you achieving your goal.

Lastly, wake up every morning and speak your goals out loud as if you've already accomplished them.

Say to yourself …

"I am healthy."

"I am successful."

"I am confident."

"I am a good father or mother."

"I am generous."

"I am kind."

"I am an amazing spouse."

"I am blessed."

Fill in the blank. "I am ______" with whatever it is you are hoping to move towards in your life.

These affirmations will help you make your dreams a reality.

Here are your key takeaways:

- Set massive goals that excite you.
- Goals should scare you because they are big, but also because they are too scary not to succeed.
- Write your goals down daily.
- Share your goals with a close friend or family member to help you stay accountable.
- Find a deeper purpose for your goals. This will help you create the desire, passion, and motivation to reach every single one.
- Wake up every morning and say "I am ..."

CHAPTER 12

Master Fear & Doubt

(STEP 5)

"Inaction breeds doubt and fear. Action breeds confidence and courage. If you want to conquer fear, do not sit home and think about it. Go out and get busy."
– Dale Carnegie

It was a beautiful summer day and I was scared out of my mind as the plane climbed toward 13,000 feet.

Out of nowhere, the plane door came open and that's when it began. The passengers started jumping out.

I was pushed toward the door and the next thing I knew, I was floating in the sky hurling towards earth. At that same moment, I felt a calm cover me as I looked out at the beautiful horizon.

Once I had finally jumped out of the plane, my fear and doubt were gone.

You see, what I didn't mention was I signed up for this experience.

Yes, I was skydiving.

All the passengers had signed up as well. Each of us were strapped to an experienced sky diver.

I'll never forget how freaked out I was on the inside before jumping out of the plane. Then, after jumping, my fear and doubt subsided.

This concept applies to other areas of our lives as well.

When I started my plan to rid myself of Crohn's, I had plenty of fear and doubt.

I asked myself:

"What if this doesn't work?"

"What if what I'm doing will make things worse?"

"Will I have to get surgery and remove my intestines, colon, or rectum?"

"How sick will the medicine make me if I must take it?"

There was lots of fear and doubt.

Fear and doubt will almost certainly be a part of your journey to success, but we must overcome it with belief and action.

Our thoughts are super powerful.

They can leave us in a tailspin of despair or lift us high into the clouds.

I had to fight past my own fear and doubt to overcome my disease. Almost everywhere I looked, I was being told I needed to be on medication for the rest of my life. That there was a 50% chance of needing some type of intestinal surgery.

If I didn't believe there was another way, and if I had listened to the majority, I would never have taken action.

Take Action

Acting and getting small or big wins will help you overcome fear and doubt too.

When I was sick and started implementing my plan, it took a while before I saw any results. Weeks would go by and nothing had changed.

Slowly however, I began to see small improvements. With each small change, I could feel my confidence grow.

Each time I would use the restroom it was a test. Somedays were very discouraging. But I didn't give up.

When I acted and my plan started working, my fear and doubt began to subside.

Small successes gave me more confidence, which encouraged more, and more action. Finally, I achieved my goal.

What Fears Are Holding You Back?

So what fears do you have?

Do you doubt yourself or the passions you want to pursue?

Do you doubt whether you can be successful?

Perhaps you have failed at a business you had to close or sell. You lost money and are scared to try again.

Is everyone around you telling you to play it safe, give up on your dreams to start a new business or a new career.

Maybe you have had a dream to move somewhere for a long time, but you feel the pressure to stay close to your friends and family. Your fears of the unknown are keeping from living somewhere amazing.

Have you had a bad past relationship? Is that experience and fear of it happening again, keeping you from falling in love with the man or woman of your dreams.

Perhaps you've let fear keep you from quitting a job that's holding you back from your true passions.

Maybe you are afraid to talk to your spouse about an issue that's keeping you from a more connected relationship.

Are you letting what others might think or say about you, keep you from your destiny?

But, what if you could have the successful business or career you've always wanted?

Or, what if you could live in a vacation destination, walking the beach every morning, sharing those moments with the man or woman of your dreams?

Well, the cure is simple. Take action my friend, and your fear and doubts will subside.

With fear and doubt out of the way, you'll have an invincible confidence that will propel you towards all your dreams.

It's that simple.

Here are your key takeaways:

- To achieve success, you'll have to overcome your fears and doubts.
- The best way to overcome fear and doubt is to take action every single day.

CHAPTER 13

Commit

(STEP 6)

"The only limit to your impact is your
imagination and commitment."
– Tony Robbins

I stood there and watched, as the rain came pouring down.

Just minutes earlier, it appeared it would be a beautiful day. That's how fast the weather changes in Iowa.

A flavor of Mark Twain's words gets quoted all the time in the Midwest.

Mark Twain said, "If you don't like the weather in New England now, just wait a few minutes."

In Iowa, people say, "If you don't like the weather in Iowa now, just wait a few minutes."

I witnessed the accuracy of this statement first hand that summer day. Unfortunately, I happened to be in my tuxedo and the start of my wedding was less than one hour away.

All the chairs had been set up in a beautiful, outdoor garden area. So much time and preparation had been put into that day.

I was nervous. The rain kept coming. At one point, it was blowing completely sideways. I closed my eyes and said a quick prayer.

And what do you know? About fifteen minutes before the start of our wedding, it stopped raining!

We rushed to get the chairs dried off, so our guests could sit down.

The wedding began, and it was amazing. My beautiful wife Natalie walked down the aisle and we've been on an incredible journey ever since.

It's been over twelve years since that day I committed to her. It remains my single biggest commitment to date. Here is the simple revelation about commitment I've discovered in those twelve years.

The more I commit, and the more we commit to each other, the better our marriage becomes. Because of this commitment to her every day and to improve myself as an individual, our relationship is better than ever.

The Power of Commitment

The power of commitment was obvious again while fighting my disease.

Early in my recovery phase, I remember once going to a famous, local barbecue restaurant. I was so tempted to order some brisket or some other delicious meat-smothered meal.

I resisted and ordered a black bean burger without a bun.

That was tough.

It took this level of commitment *day after day* until my disease was gone.

In the beginning, every day seemed like a bad day with this disease. I didn't see any results for some time. I tried several things at first that didn't seem to have results, but I kept persisting until I found what worked.

Are You Committed?

Can you imagine a time when you have fully committed to achieving success?

Were you able to accomplish your goals?

Did you maintain discipline and continue fighting even after some things didn't work?

I have a feeling that if you did commit yourself fully, every day, you succeeded.

Here is another Grant Cardone quote I love:

> *"Success tends to bless those who are most committed to giving it the most attention."*

Success is not a mystery. You must fully commit.

Then, once you've committed, you must take action, day after day. True success demands persistence and discipline over time.

If I had implemented my plan to eliminate Crohn's for just a few days or a week, I would not have been successful.

There were so many days I wanted to eat food I knew wasn't good for me, but I resisted. I was very disciplined. Each day I decided I would stay on course and not give up.

Success is only for those who persist and have the discipline to do so.

So, are you ready to commit? Are you ready to go all in every day?

I believe each of us has a more amazing life waiting for us if we simply commit.

Decide, right now, to commit yourself each day to live the BIG LIFE you were meant for.

Then, re-commit yourself every morning to the same. Every time you get tempted to give up or delay, so NO! Today, I am committed to my dreams and nothing will stand in my way!

Here are your key takeaways:

- Fully commit to the success you desire. Go all in.
- When times get tough or something doesn't work out, keep trying. Stay disciplined and persistent until you achieve your desired result.
- You need to commit, then recommit to achieve your goals every single day.

CHAPTER 14

Never Stop Learning

(STEP 7)

"The best investment you can make is in yourself."
– Warren Buffet

It was 4am and our alarm went off. My brother and I woke up and went downstairs. We opened the front door and started bringing in piles of stacked newspapers.

Then, we began to fold and place rubber bands around them, getting the papers ready for the morning delivery.

Yes, my thirteen-year-old brother and I, just ten at the time, were paper boys.

We hopped on our bikes full of papers and went out to deliver that morning like any other day.

Most days, it was foggy and a bit dangerous for youngsters like us. We even delivered along a 5-mile busy stretch of road, on the bad side of town. Looking back, I'm not sure how our parents let us take that job.

We both survived, so that's the important thing.

My brother and I were addicted to video games. We used all the extra money we earned from the paper route to purchase more games.

One morning, I was delivering my last paper and was relieved to be finished. I hopped on my bike and started pedaling.

That's when I saw it.

A huge Great Dane running straight towards me. I pedaled as fast as I could to try and outrun it. But, it was no use.

The Great Dane caught up to me quickly and I was scared out of my mind.

This dog was huge!

I remember it running right alongside me, standing just as tall or taller than I was.

Luckily, I got away. It must have gotten bored of chasing me.

My brother and I headed back to the house and watched some morning cartoons. Then we went back to bed to get some rest before school.

We woke up around 9:30am or 10am to start our school day. I know what you're thinking. School doesn't start at that time, that's too late.

Well, you're right.

Traditional school doesn't begin at 9:30am or 10am, but homeschool at my house did.

You see, I had been homeschooling since second grade, and loved it. I had so much freedom.

We could start late, spend a few hours on actual school work, and then I could do whatever I wanted.

One of the key skills I learned while homeschooling was the ability to figure things out on my own. Yes, my mom was around to help, but I honed the skill of research and teaching myself what I needed and wanted to learn.

This skill has been one of my greatest assets, even to this day. It's helped me to breeze through high school and college. It's helped me in my career.

This skill also saved my life when I began getting symptoms of my disease.

Once again, I went into research mode trying to figure out what was wrong with me and how I could fix it.

As I've attempted to mature as an individual, I now understand *research and continual learning are essential to success.*

For us to succeed, we need to encourage the curiosity of knowledge.

It can be deceiving to think we have it all figured out or have heard it all before. But, I've found, the more I learn, the more I understand, how little I know.

Each nugget of gold I find makes me want to find another.

Gold Rush

One popular show on these days is Gold Rush.

I love this reality TV show. It documents the lives and businesses of gold diggers in the Alaskan Yukon trying to strike it rich.

These individuals endure extreme weather and work conditions all for the love of gold. They have gold fever.

While I've never had gold fever, I am hungry for knowledge. I am excited to find hidden nuggets of golden information.

Once you begin the path of self-development like you're already on, it can be addicting.

But that's a great thing.

You see, if we want success, we need to become the people who deserve the success we achieve.

As I battled my disease, I continued learning as much as I could on how I could conquer it. The more I learned and acted on the information, I became the person who deserved the success I achieved.

So, don't stopped learning.

Don't give up researching the solutions to your life.

Keep learning and feeding your hunger for knowledge.

Continue investing in yourself like you have by reading this book. Never believe the lie you have it all figured out. Stay humble and hungry for knowledge.

Here are your key takeaways:

- Invest in yourself.
- Become an individual who is willing to research on your own and seek to find answers.
- Become the person worthy of the success you desire by continually learning and improving yourself.

CHAPTER 15

Dominate Your Health

(STEP 8)

*"If you don't have your health,
you don't have anything."*
– Chuck Pagano

It was 6am and I was awoken by a knock at the door.

At the time, I was going to college and living with my grandpa in his Long Beach, California home.

Who was it, I thought?

I rolled out of bed and opened the door. It was my friend Gil.

Before I could ask why he had woken me up so early, he said, *"The waves are breaking, let's go surfing."*

I said OK, if we're back before my 10am class.

Gil said, no problem, and I threw my board and wetsuit into the back of his car and we took off.

This became a regular habit. Then, when the waves were epic, you guessed it, I didn't make it back to class.

The problem was, living in southern California, near Huntington Beach, the waves were amazing all the time.

While it made it more difficult to get the grades I wanted, it was well worth it. I had a blast!

My grandpa, Marcos, very kindly let me stay with him while finishing my math degree.

He was a big believer in education.

He came from a poor Hispanic background with many siblings. He was one of only a few in his family who graduated from high school and perhaps the only one to get a college degree.

He received his degree in aerospace engineering from the University of Southern California.

Quite an accomplishment, especially considering his roots.

One day, after class, I received some bad news, my grandpa had cancer. It turns out he had been fighting it for quite some time.

I remember very clearly one of the last conversations I had with him.

He quoted Pagano and said, "If you don't have your health, you don't have anything."

A month or two later, my grandpa had passed.

I was reminded once again of Pagano and my grandpa's words as I received the diagnosis of a *"chronic"* disease.

Without our health, none of us have much.

If health is not currently your focus, it will be eventually. Even without a chronic disease, when we aren't taking care of our bodies, we lack energy and cannot be our best.

I'm not saying I know the exact cause of my disease, but I believe the way I was treating my body was a major contribution.

Eventually, our health will catch up to all of us. If you aren't treating your body right, it will let you know in numerous, adverse ways. When we're healthy, eating well, exercising regularly, and sleeping great, we'll have the energy and clarity of thought to succeed.

Four Keys to Amazing Health

Four years prior to writing this book, my wife and I owned and operated a surf inspired gym in Huntington Beach, California.

This was before I was diagnosed with Crohn's. I applied some this knowledge and experience to heal myself and I want to offer some of this same advice to you now.

If you have any type of bowel disorder (Irritable Bowel Disease or Irritable Bowel Syndrome), pay close attention. However, this advice is for everyone seeking to improve their health today.

The recipe is simple, but very powerful.

If you apply these tips to your life, you're certain to succeed with your health.

However, I must state, I am not a doctor, and everyone body is different. So, please consult your physician for all medical advice and treatment related to your personal health.

Here are the four categories of better health I'll be covering.

1. Exercise
2. Sleep
3. Stress
4. Diet

All the above are very important, but I'll spend the most time on diet, since this has had the biggest impact on my road to recovery.

Don't Forget to Exercise

"To enjoy the glow of good health, you must exercise."

– Gene Tunney

Ok, we all know exercise is good for us. We all know we should exercise but let me share what's worked for me.

When I ran my gym, we focused on group fitness. We felt that group environment helped better motivate and keep people accountable. Our core belief was helping others get fit in sixty days or less. We did this with classes that were just thirty minutes long.

Most members would work out with us three to five days a week.

That's it.

We had some amazing results with this formula and so can you. The key is consistency which I believe group fitness helps with.

During some 60-day sessions we would offer our members a $1000 prize for the individual with the greatest transformation.

This was a great motivator for our members to give it their all.

In my journey to health and fitness I've had my ups and downs. When I've had my greatest results, I've always had something pushing me; some type of reward I would receive if I reached a certain level of fitness or health.

This was also true with my disease. I had huge motivation to get healthy and fit.

So, find something to motivate you, whether that's competition or a trip to look good on. Find your why!

Then, be consistent.

You don't have to work out for an hour or two or three hours a day. Thirty minutes is enough, especially if you're pushing yourself. Quality over quantity.

Also, make sure you aren't solely focused on cardio. I've seen many favor a cardio workout, myself included, but building muscle is critical to a fit body.

Muscle burns calories while resting. So, the more muscle you have, the more calories you'll burn throughout the day without the extra effort. You'll also be much stronger.

So, I highly recommend joining a group fitness program. Look for a local program that incorporates strength training with classes that last 30 to 60 minutes. Make sure to workout three to five days a week, and you'll be golden.

Get Some Sleep

"Sleep is a time of intense neurological activity – a rich time of renewal, memory consolidation, brain and neurochemical cleansing, and cognitive maintenance. Properly appraised, our sleeping time is as valuable a commodity as the time we are awake. In fact, getting the right amount of sleep enhances the quality of every minute we spend with our eyes open."
– Arianna Huffington

Sleep is critical to success and our health. Without proper sleep, we cannot live healthy, thriving lives.

Many of us take sleeping pills to wind ourselves down at the end of the day. Then, to wake up in the morning or during the day, we drink coffee or consume energy drinks.

This unnatural cycle feeds itself and increases our risk of major health problems.

Here are just some of the risks from sleep deprivation:

- Heart disease
- Heart attack
- Heart failure
- Irregular heartbeat
- High blood pressure
- Diabetes
- Spreading of cancer

- Infertility
- Higher stress levels
- Lowers sex drive

Sleep deprivation has become a major problem for many in America.

Arianna Huffington also speaks about how sleep deprivation has become a factor in job burnout:

> *"Thirty percent of employed Americans now report getting six hours of sleep or less per night, and nearly 70 percent describe their sleep as insufficient. Getting by on less than six hours of sleep is one of the biggest factors in job burnout."*

If you want success in your life, with your career, and with your health, make sleep a priority.

Sleep is an area of health that I believe is very underrated. I know I've not given it as much importance as the other areas of health.

I was always a night owl. I tended to stay up until midnight most nights. Then, forced to get up early for work or my kids, I would wake up grumpy and lacking energy the next day.

Having four kids now has encouraged me to get to bed early.

Getting a great night sleep has dramatically improved my attitude, clarity of mind, and connection with my family. I am far more balanced and productive during my day.

I want to encourage you to do the same. Try to get at least *seven to nine hours* of sleep each night. With a great night's rest, you'll live a healthy, energetic, productive, and balanced life.

Manage Your Stress

"The greatest weapon against stress is our ability

to choose one thought over another."

– William James

When I got sick, I was very stressed out. I was eating poorly and wasn't exercising very much. I had a lot on my mind and worried far too much.

I truly believe stress was a major contributor to my health problems.

As I fought my disease over the last few years, I learned a lot.

Here are some simple recommendations for managing your stress.

1. Get your mind right
2. Exercise
3. Get a great night sleep
4. Hit up the steam

Get your mind right

Make *Conquest* and the ten success habits found in this book part of your belief system. Listen to positive books on tape or podcasts.

When your mind is in the right place, you'll be able to handle anything life throws your way.

Exercise

When I exercise, I feel great. I have more confidence, energy, and life. My stress seems to melt away after a good workout and yours will too.

Get a great night sleep

Lack of sleep has been shown to increase the stress hormone cortisol. But, when we get a great night sleep, we have more patience and don't let small things get to us so easily.

Even when something big comes along, a great night sleep will better prepare our mind and body to handle it.

Hit Up the Steam

Releasing the toxins by relaxing in a hot bath or steam room are great for stress relief. It just feels great. I also recommend putting some Epson salt and eucalyptus drops in the bath to open your lungs and help you breathe.

You will most certainly sleep better, feel more relaxed, and detoxify your body.

Simple Lifestyle Changes

Did you know that heart disease is the number one cause of death in the world? A reported 633,842 people died from heart disease in 2014.

This number makes me very sad.

Heart disease is almost always lifestyle driven. In most cases, it's preventable and treatable by simple lifestyle changes like better diet or by quitting smoking.

So, whether you have Crohn's disease, heart problems, or just want more energy throughout your day, here are the health tips that saved my life.

Elimination, Supplements, & Detox

During my research to uncover a solution to my gut issues, I kept coming across Dr. Hyman's content online. Dr. Hyman is a *New York Times* bestselling author and specializes in functional medicine.

Functional medicine is a holistic type of alternative medicine.

I was excited about Dr. Hyman's approach, because traditional thinking was to treat the disease with expensive medicines with many side effects.

Dr. Hyman had some great articles on his blog speaking directly about IBS and other gut issues:

- <u>5 Simple Steps to Cure IBS Without Drugs</u>
- <u>Powerful Strategies to Eliminate IBS and Other Gut Issues</u>

Articles such as these encouraged me to start an elimination diet. Here are some of the things I initially eliminated from my diet:

- Dairy
- Gluten
- Yeast
- Eggs
- Corn
- Soy
- Peanuts

- Sugar
- Caffeine
- Alcohol

So, first I recommend eliminating anything you eat now that you know doesn't make you feel well.

I have mixed feelings about the accuracy of allergy tests, but you might want to do some additional research and consider taking one.

Otherwise, use the bulleted list above to remove the bad stuff from your diet.

Keep in mind, this elimination diet was only temporary until my symptoms were relieved. Today, I enjoy many foods and drinks that contain these ingredients.

Next, I was attracted to Dr. Hyman's *Super Simple Diet*.

While I wasn't trying to lose weight, this diet also focused on inflammation reduction, detox, and stress management.

This is Dr. Hyman's older book so you may want to check out his latest program, *The Blood Sugar Solution 10 Day Detox Diet*.

Dr. Hyman's program helped right away. Both of these programs offer great results in a minimal amount of time, 7 to 10 days or less.

The *Super Simple Diet* encouraged specific supplements as well. While I didn't follow the exact instructions, I was able to achieve great results with similar supplements below. Most of these I purchased through Amazon:

- **Multi-Vitamin** - Vitality Organic Life Vitamins
- **Probiotics** – Hyperbiotics PRO-15 Probiotics
- **Vitamin C** – Metagenics Ultra Potent-C

- <u>Omega 3s</u> – <u>Vital Choice Wild Alaskan Salmon Oil</u>
- <u>Shake Powder</u> - <u>Shakeology</u>

Become a Pegan

What's a Pegan you might ask?

A Pegan diet is a blend between the Paleo diet and Vegan diet.

You've most likely heard of these diets. Dr. Hyman coined the phrase Pegan.

You can read all about this diet in his article *Why I am a Pegan – or Paleo-Vegan – and Why You Should Be Too*!

Here are some key guidelines Dr. Hyman provides:

- Eat the right fats, like nuts and avocados. Also, saturated fat from grass fed or sustainably raised animals is ok.
- Avoid dairy (cheese, for example).
- Avoid gluten (bread, for example).
- Eat beans infrequently.
- Meat should be a side dish, not the main course.
- Eat sugar sparingly as an occasional treat.
- Eat fish low in mercury, for example, wild salmon and sardines.
- Vegetables and fruit should consist of 75% of your diet.

Quite the opposite of the traditional American diet, right?

That last bullet might jump out at you. When I first read I should be consuming that many fruits and vegetables, I felt overwhelmed. But, I didn't give up. I needed to find a solution.

Sick, Fat, and Nearly Dead

If you haven't seen it already, you must watch the documentary, *Sick, Fat, and Nearly Dead*.

In this film, Joe Cross attempts to regain his health through juicing. He juiced for 60 days straight. The results he gained were amazing including losing 78 lbs. and almost eliminated all medication.

I remembered this film when I got sick and thought, *"maybe I can heal myself with juicing too and will be able to consume the amounts of fruits and vegetables I need."*

Additionally, some online forum members were discussing amazing results by going on a strict juicing diet.

So, that's when I decided to become a juicing pagan!

I would consume the necessary fruits and vegetables as part of Dr. Hyman's program, by juicing.

Juicing Basics

So, what is juicing and why should you juice?

Juicing is the process of extracting the juices from fruits and vegetables. The juices contain most of the nutrients, so you get a high dose of healthiness when juicing.

Juicing has helped me enjoy fruits and vegetables far more.

As Dr. Hyman recommended, 75% of our food should come from fruits and vegetables. Again, I have a difficult time consuming that many fruits and veggies. The solution for me has been juicing. Juicing also retains the nutrients far more than if you were to cook your vegetables.

While not necessary, I recommend buying a high-quality juicer to extract the juice.

Personally, I bought a Super Angel, one of the very best. I spent over $1300 on this juicer. You don't have to spend this much. You can buy some juicers on Amazon for as little as $50 or even less.

But, be careful. If you're serious about juicing, *I recommend getting the best juicer you can afford*. Here is why.

There's a massive difference in the amounts of juice extracted from one juicer to another. Also, some pulp can be found in the juice from lower quality juicers.

A good rule of thumb is if your pulp is wet, your juicer is not doing the best job at extracting all the juice. Since the cost of fruits and vegetables can add up if juicing on a regular basis, getting the juicer that extracts the most juice makes sense, right?

Of course, it does. Otherwise, you'll just be spending much more on produce in the long run.

After watching numerous juicer comparison videos on YouTube, it was obvious. Even many of the top-rated juicers on Amazon did not come close to the Super Angel.

The Super Angel extracted 2x, 3x, 5x, 10x or more juice.

Over time, it's going to cost you far more to purchase more fruits and vegetables than investing in a good quality juicer up front.

Now, don't confuse juicing with buying juice from your local grocery store. Most juices in the store have far less nutritional value since most are pasteurized and oxidized.

A pro and con of juicing is it removes the pulp or fiber from the juice. There are many digestive, metabolic, and cardiovascular benefits of fiber. Soluble fiber can also help reduce constipation. Constipation was not my problem however. Just the opposite in fact.

So, in my case, removing pulp was a very good thing. Without soluble fiber, my digestive system had a break from processing food and nutrients were absorbed more quickly.

Remember, if you want some fiber in your juice, simply put some of the pulp back into the juice from the pulp extracted through the juicing process.

Blending Basics

An alternative to juicing is *blending with a blender*. I use a combination of both in my diet.

There are some key differences between juicing and blending that are important to note. The four big differences are fiber, taste, type, and quantity.

Fiber

With blending, all the fiber is kept within the juice or smoothie. However, if desired, fiber can be added back into juice from the pulp that's been extracted.

Taste

The taste of a pure juice and vegetables that have been blended with the pulp are far different.

For example, I love juicing broccoli. But blend broccoli and it just doesn't taste the same. Once you start blending and juicing, you'll discover your favorite fruits and vegetables to blend and juice.

The key for me was to make fruits and vegetables 75% of my diet, like Dr. Hyman recommends.

Type

Some types of fruits and vegetables are un-juiceable. They simply cannot be juiced.

A couple of examples are bananas and avocados. While I love both foods, I am unable to juice them.

They can be blended however. Just add some water and blend to make an awesome smoothie.

Nutrients

Lastly, let's talk nutrients.

Pay attention here. This by far has had the greatest impact on my health and Crohn's *Conquest.*

Since most of the vitamins and minerals come from the juice of the fruit and vegetable, I lean towards juicing.

Understanding this allowed me to focus on juicing where I could absorb higher levels of nutrients more quickly.

While cost and hunger must be considered, you can juice and consume far more kale than you could consume by blending for example. The fiber creates a larger drink to consume. However, because of the fiber, less fruits or vegetables are consumed within the same size drink. So, less nutrients are consumed as well.

We must recognize the benefits of pulp and fiber however, so the balance of juicing and blending should be a personal choice and dependent on your goals.

I do recommend getting both a high-quality blender and juicer. I've used the same Blendtec blender for over 5 years. Vitamix also has a great product.

Avoid Pesticides

To reduce pesticide consumption, I highly recommend eating organic fruits and vegetables if you can afford them, especially when the fruit or vegetable does not have a hard skin layer.

A good example of a hard skin layer would be a banana. It's not as important to get organic bananas in my opinion. However, if eating leafy greens like kale or spinach, do your best to go organic.

What You Should Juice & Blend

So, what should you juice and blend?

This is personal choice. You need to consider what you enjoy, what you will drink, and may differ based on your personal health.

I do encourage you to step out and try some new things. Some juices are an acquired taste. Others, I don't love, but drink because I know how good they are for me. For example, I almost always make a ginger shot along with my primary juice.

It's not the greatest feeling right away, but it does feel nice and warm going down. Ginger is a super food and it's been a key ingredient in healing myself.

I also juice lots of kale, spinach, beets, carrots, broccoli, cucumber and apples. It's been easier to find organic versions of these at my local store. Beyond their health benefits, that's why I juice these specific fruits and vegetables.

For blending, I'll add high quality, US produced spirulina and vegetable-based protein powder to my drinks. I currently use Sun Warriors Organic Plant Based Protein Powder. I tend to blend kale and spinach like juicing, but not many of the other fruits or vegetables I mentioned.

Instead, I'll add more fruits like bananas, pineapple, mangoes, and berries.

These tend to be easier to find frozen, so they make great smoothie ingredients.

You'll be able to find some great juice recipes online as well on sites like Juicerecipes.com.

Enjoy the juice and your health.

The Conquest Health Challenge

So, are you sick? Do you lack energy?

Perhaps you aren't aware of how sick you are. When our lifestyle has been a certain way for a long time, we get used to being sick, tired, or lethargic. It becomes our new normal.

Let me challenge you today to spend a week focused on your health.

Here is what I want you to do:

1. Commit to <u>Dr. Hymans 10 Day Detox</u> or <u>Joe Cross's Reboot Program</u>. Don't wait, start one of these programs in the next couple weeks.
2. Commit to getting seven to nine hours of sleep this week. If you are already doing that, great. Well done! But, if not, then make this a priority this week and see how it feels.
3. Spend a two to three days this week taking a hot bath. If you have a gym membership with a spa, then relax in there. If there is a steam room, then jump in there also. Use this time to reflect on what you learned in this book. Get your mind right and ready for success.
4. (Optional) If you really want to take your health to the next level, jump on full time as a Juicing Pagan.

I guarantee by taking the steps, you'll feel amazing, have far more energy, and be on your way to fantastic health.

Here are your key takeaways:

- The four keys to excellent health are: regular exercise, stress management, enough sleep, and the right diet.
- The right diet was critical in conquering Crohns.
- For a proper diet, start by eliminating bad foods from your diet and add supplements.
- 75% of our diet should consist of fruits and vegetables.
- To consume this many fruits and vegetables, I highly recommend adding juicing and blending to your daily eating routines.
- Take the Conquest Health Challenge. I dare you!

CHAPTER 16

Let Faith Set You Free

(STEP 9)

"I believe if you keep your faith, you keep your trust, you keep
the right attitude, if you're grateful, you'll see God open up new
doors."
– Joel Osteen

One normal day, when I was twelve years old,   I was home with my mother.

She was working on a wood project of some kind and asked me if I could help her out. She needed a piece of wood cut and asked if I would cut it on our table saw.

I said, *"sure, no problem mom."*

I grabbed the piece of wood and took it into the garage where our table saw was. Our table saw was very old and a bit broken. A nail needed to be inserted into the broken on/off switch then moved to the right, to turn it on, and to the left to turn it off.

I was always a bit nervous when using it, especially since there weren't any safety guards. However, I didn't think much of it at the time since I had used it many times before.

I turned on the saw and began sliding the piece of wood through the blade, cutting the wood. I remember telling myself, keep your hands away from the blade.

I slid the wood all the way through and breathed a sigh of relief. Then, I turned off the table saw and grabbed the piece of wood my mom needed.

I took a few steps back toward the door that led back into the house. Then, I stopped and began to replay the wood cut in mind.

If you've ever cut a piece of wood, you know that the saw will make a distinct buzzing sound just as the wood is finished being cut. Well, I remember thinking to myself, I heard two of those sounds, one right after the other, not just one, like I should have.

That's when I looked down at my hand. After seeing a bunch of blood, I realized, I had cut my thumb completely off!

I yelled frantically for my mom. She came rushing into the garage, realized what I had done, and called 911.

Soon, an ambulance came and rushed me to the hospital. Sitting there, waiting to find out what would happen next, a great peace came over me. It was the greatest sense of peace I had ever experienced. I remember the nurses mentioning how calm I was.

This peace was not a coincidence. You see, even at a young age, I had a strong faith in God. I was praying the entire time, recognizing that God would take care of me and that everything would be alright.

I was eventually driven about two hours away, to a hospital in San Francisco. Here, they had some highly skilled micro surgeons who would attempt to reattach my thumb.

How cool is that!

I remember saying one last prayer before the anesthesia kicked in, then I was out.

After a few hours in surgery, the doctors came out to speak with my parents. They told them they didn't think they would be able to reattach my thumb because they were unable to find the necessary veins and arteries. My dad spoke to them and asked if they would try one last time.

So, they did.

A few hours later, the surgery was over, and they had found the veins and arteries to reattach my thumb!

I recovered in the hospital over the next couple weeks and am so grateful and blessed to still have my thumb today.

While my relationship with God has had its ups and downs, my faith in God has always remained. Again, when I was facing health issues with my gut, I prayed, *"God, it's all in your hands."*

Again, God took care of me and I am so blessed to be healthier than ever, today.

With faith, you won't have to handle the trials and tribulations of life all by yourself. Moreover, new and amazing opportunities will open to you like never before.

God Will Always Be There for You

Perhaps you once had faith but have walked from it. Maybe, God was once a big part of your life, but you stopped praying or going to church.

Let me just say from personal experience, God still loves you, wants to bless you, and have a relationship with you.

You see, I grew up in the church. I attended Sunday school every week, went to church camp, and read my bible regularly. In high school, I was the bible club president for three years. I even helped lead worship for a local church and their children's ministry.

However, a few years after high school, my long-time high school girlfriend and I broke up. I was tore up. Something inside gave up on faith and God for some time.

It took a long while, but I feel back on track again. In all that time, God did not give up on me. He never left me. He was always there and will always be there for me.

He will always be there for you too.

It doesn't matter if stopped praying or if you never started, God is there with open arms, ready to accept you just as you are.

Mr. Osteen

I want to share a Youtube clip about faith from an amazing pastor named Joel Osteen.

Here is the link:

https://www.youtube.com/watch?v=5JjEt2EJI14

Joel Osteen is a hugely popular televangelist based in Houston, Texas. He is the author of seven New York Times Best-selling books. His sermons are seen in over 100 countries with over 20 million viewers a month.

Now, you may not believe in God or have faith in much. But, I challenge you. If you simply open your mind to the possibility that you don't know something, perhaps you'll give God and faith a chance.

Or, maybe you walked away from God for a bit and gone your own way. Perhaps Joel's message will inspire you to put your life in God's hands once again.

With such popularity and momentum, surely Joel has something worth hearing right?

Please, give Joel's video on faith a chance, and I know it will inspire you. Perhaps something will resonate within you. Something that has been locked deep inside for a long time.

If you are a man or woman of faith, Joel's words will most certainly encourage you. So please, take just a little time to listen to Joel's Faith Video and his Youtube channel for more inspirational videos.

I pray these words and Joel's, will reach your heart and inspire you to do great things in life.

Here are your key takeaways:

- God will always be there for you, no matter what.
- Don't live life alone. Let God lift your burdens.
- Healing and blessings are found through faith.
- Get inspired to do big things by listing to Joel's Faith Video.

CHAPTER 17

Leave a Lasting Legacy

(STEP 10)

"If you would not be forgotten as soon as you are dead, either write something worth reading, or do something worth writing about."
– Benjamin Franklin

In recent years, I've been on a journey of self-development and improvement.

My wife, Natalie and I have become big fans of Grant Cardone.

His books and multitude of Facebook live events have inspired us to reach for our dreams at all costs.

One day, Grant offered free tickets to an entrepreneurial conference called Thrive, in exchange for purchasing tickets to his Growth Con conference.

My wife took him up on the offer, and at the end of September, we were off to Las Vegas.

The conference was amazing.

One presenter made me think hard about my own legacy.

The speaker started a conversation with a man in the audience.

The audience member wanted to start a music production company to provide an amazing service for struggling musicians. But he was afraid to give up his current income stream to do it.

He didn't enjoy his current work, but still hesitated, and was fearful to take that leap.

As the presenter tried to persuade the man to follow his passions, he said, *"Just imagine the lives of all the people you will not get to help, if you don't start your music company."*

That hit home for me.

I had so many thoughts as I left Vegas, Sunday afternoon, October 1st, 2017.

We woke up the next morning to discover my wife and I had missed the deadliest mass shooting in modern US history, by just 7 hours.

The shooting made me question my legacy.

"What if that had been my wife and I, caught in the line of fire?"

"What if we were still in Vegas when the shooting started?"

I had similar thoughts of my legacy when I was first diagnosed with Crohn's. Being diagnosed with a potential, life threatening, *"incurable disease"*, was a huge wake up call.

What was my legacy to be? Was this my demise?

Now I realize it was not, but my mortality became clear. Each of us will die. But how will we be remembered?

It's never too early or late to start leaving your legacy.

If you're *"young"*, you might believe you're too young to make a difference or leave a legacy.

However, Mark Zuckerberg was just 19 years old when he launched Facebook.

If you're *"old"*, you might believe it's too late to make an impact or to change.

Julia Child didn't start her PBS cooking show until age 51. Colonel Sanders started KFC at age 65.

So, you must realize, age is just an excuse.

Yes, time is after us all and our time is limited. However, since you're reading this, you still have time.

Time for what you might ask?

To tell your story. To give the world your very best. To find your passion and inspire others. To live a big life. To leave your legacy.

I believe each of us wants to be remembered and in the very best way possible.

This self-reflection and discovery has led me to the opening quote by Benjamin Franklin and writing this book.

He states, if we want to leave a lasting legacy, we need to:

1. Do something worth writing about
2. Or, write something worth reading

Doing Something Worth Writing About

There are hundreds and thousands of individuals we only know of now, because they did something incredible.

Their lives have influenced us somehow. Their names have gone down in the history books. Some of these individuals are still alive and others passed away.

But they all hold one thing in common, they have left a lasting legacy.

My hope is the elements of *Conquest* you have learned in this book, will help you do something worth writing about.

With these habits, you'll have the courage to believe in your big, scary goals. You'll be able to overcome fears and doubt with action while fully committing to your cause.

If you want to be remembered in a big way, you must set massive goals and take massive action. Keep learning and discovering what excites you. Grow healthy habits. I have no doubt these ten elements of *Conquest* will strengthen you to leave your legacy.

Write Something Worth Reading

I am not a writer. I studied mathematics and computers in college.

However, I recently discovered the power of writing and have embraced it. I believe it is one of the very best ways to tell my story and to have a greater impact on this world. To help others and live forever.

So how did I write this book without being a writer? I just started writing. That's it.

As I began writing, I gained more and more confidence that I could write a book.

I also discovered I didn't have to write a 400 or 500-page book. This made the task far less daunting. Most readers these days want less, more concise information. Yes, you can write a larger book, but there's nothing wrong with even a 15-page book if the information is good.

Another trick I found was a way to write without writing. While I did type a lot of this book, some sections were constructed by simply speaking into my computer microphone and recorded my voice with a free application called Audacity. Then, with free voice recognition software, I turned the recording into written words.

So, if you prefer speaking over writing, you can simply take your outline and start talking about each point while recording. Then, turn the recording into text. It's as easy as that.

Another question you might have is, what should I write about?

Well, that takes some digging, but I recommend writing what you're passionate about. Go back to Chapter 9 and make sure you understand your desires and passions.

Writing a "How To" book is also easy to do. So, if you have something you're good at and something you're passionate about, there's your book. Just take your readers on a journey from start to end on how they will get from point A to point B.

Lastly, if you need additional help writing, need a coach, or a program to follow, I've created all of this at writeabookuniversity.com.

I'll help YOU write, publish, and market an amazing book.

In addition to writing books myself, I decided that helping others write a book is the second-best way I can help the world be a better place. I want to help as many people as I can write their stories and help other people. By doing so, I'll be helping far more people and touching more lives than I ever could on my own.

So, don't wait to leave your legacy. Write a book, help others, and live forever.

Here are your key takeaways:

- To leave a lasting legacy, do something worth writing about, or write something worth reading.
- To do something worth writing about, use the ten elements of *Conquest*. You're never too young or old to dream big and do big things.
- Write a book to leave your legacy. Write about what you're passionate about and help others.
- Go to <u>writeabookuniversity.com</u> for more help on writing a book.

CHAPTER 18

We Are What We Remember

(PRO STEP)

"Memory is all we are. Moments and feelings, captured in amber, strung on filaments of reason. Take a man's memories and you take all of him. Chip away a memory at a time and you destroy him as surely as if you hammered nail after nail through his skull."
– Mark Lawrence

Ok, I'm going to tell you a crazy story, but just stick in there. I promise there's a purpose behind it.

Just imagine, walking into your *home living room*. You grab the remote and turn on the **Discovery** Channel. You see some wild animals on the screen playing **disc** frisbee, then boom. The TV Explodes! (Discovery)

The explosion knocks you into the *kitchen*. You hit the *fridge* hard and turn around as it transforms into a big **dessert with tires** for sprinkles. (Desire)

The explosion has made a huge hole in the *side of your home*. A large gust of wind blows in some **bees and leaves** that begin swarming you and the dessert. (Believe)

The bees pick up the dessert and drop it on the *oven*. The bees start eating the dessert and begin growing **bigger and bigger** and you scream because you're so **scared**. They turn into football players, roll you into a ball, and kick you through a field **goal** post. (Big Scary Goals)

You land inside the *dishwasher*, right onto your **ear**. A **flower** starts growing out of your ear. Then a **dog** with a body like a **trout** starts eating the flowers. The dishwasher turns into an **auction**. The dog with a trout body is **auctioning** off all your dishes. (Fear, Doubt, & Action)

You run out of the *kitchen* into the *dining room*. On the *dining room table* is a **chocolate covered baseball mitt**. (Commit)

You pick up the mitt which holds a chocolate covered ball. You throw the ball and it heads right for a **leather covered urn** and knocks it over, spilling all the ashes. (Learn)

You sprint out of the dining room into your *bedroom*, but it's on fire and looks like **hell**. You throw buckets of vegetables on the fire to put it out. (Health)

You run into the *hall* outside your bedroom and look at the *pictures on the wall*. All your family photos have turned into **figure eights**. (Faith)

You head toward the *bathroom* and on your way, you lift your **leg and fart. The gas** fills the room and starts the fire up again. (Legacy)

You take your magic wand and begin to pull **memories** out of your head as a last resort to put the fire out. The memories sweep *through the room* and extinguish the fire. (Memory)

Memory Techniques

So, what was all that you might ask.

Well, since this chapter is titled remember, you might have guessed that we used a visual story to remember the ten elements of *Conquest*.

Now, I'm not a memory expert, but I've read plenty of books and used these techniques in my own life to increase my memory dramatically.

When I was back in high school, I would use techniques like this to memorize speech outlines for presentations, essay outlines for history tests, and much more.

I believe memories are so important. It's why I've included this chapter. In fact, without techniques like this, we do not remember much. According to Edgar Dale's cone of experience, we only retain 10% of what we read.

So, if you want to retain more knowledge, here is one technique you can use.

To create a medium-term memory, you must associate what you're trying to remember, with a long-term memory. Short-term memory plus long-term memory equals medium-term memory.

Our mind is great at seeing images. If you close your eyes and think of the word dog, for example, what do you see?

A dog, right!

Well, what I did in the story above, was break apart key words related to the ten elements of *Conquest* plus memory. I turned these words into more memorable, visual objects, and tied them to your house, which should be in your long-term memory.

We also better remember things that bring on emotions like fear, excitement, and joy. So, our stories should include those elements as well.

I've bolded all the keywords in the story that relate to the elements of *Conquest* and italicized some objects I considered part of my long-term memory. Here is a summary of the elements and objects again below.

The sequence is as follows: Part a | Part b | Part c

Part a: *Conquest* Element to Remember

Part b: Long Term Memory Image(s)

Part c: Short Term Memory Image(s)

- Discovery | Living Room | TV on with Discovery Channel and animals playing disk frisbee.
- Desire | Kitchen | Big Dessert with Tire Sprinkles
- Believe | Living Room | Bees and Leaves
- Big, Scary Goals | Kitchen Oven | Bees Grow Bigger, Scream, Field Goal Posts
- Fear, Doubt & Action | Kitchen Dishwasher | Flowers growing from ears, Dog with Trout Body, & Auction.
- Commit | Dining Room | Chocolate Covered Baseball Mitt
- Learn | Dining Room | Leather Covered Urn
- Health | Bedroom | Fire, Hell, and Vegetables

- Faith | Hall | Figure Eight Pictures
- Legacy | Bathroom | Leg, Fart, Gas
- Memory (Pro Tip) | Bedroom | Magic Wand to Pull Memories Out of Your Mind

One last thing to remember: using your own objects and places in your stories is very helpful as they are already part of your long-term memory. So, you could revise the story I've created with your own objects to make it more memorable.

You'll want to review these stories on a regular basis to turn those medium-term memories into long-term memories.

With this story and tools, however, you have a framework to remember the ten elements of *Conquest* and almost anything else.

Remember Names

Names, as most know, are very important to remember. The one word that's probably the most important to any individual is their name.

So, when we forget a name after being introduced or not having seen someone for a long time, it doesn't feel so good.

Have you ever forgotten a name?

Sure you have. We all have.

So, here's a quick way to remember people's names. When you're introduced, take the most prominent feature on someone's face (eyes, nose, ears, etc.) and break their name apart into more visual objects.

Let's take my name, Aaron, for example.

I feel a prominent feature of mine are my protruding ears.

So, let's start by breaking my name apart into a couple more visual words.

Imagine, ears that grow legs and start running.

This fits in perfect with ears being my prominent feature as well.

So, you could remember my name by seeing my face and then my ears. Then picturing my ears growing legs and running so fast it carries me into the air and helps me fly.

The next time you see me, you would get that image in your mind and be reminded that my name is Aaron (Ears Running).

I hope this trick makes it easier and more fun to remember names.

Happy remembering!

Here are your key takeaways:

- We are what we remember.
- To remember well, we must associate what we want to remember with our long-term memory to create a medium-term memory.
- Break words into visual objects and build those into a story tied to long term memories.
- Review stories on a regular basis to turn medium-term memories into long-term memories.
- Remember names, they are the most important words to any individual.

CHAPTER 19

What's Holding You Back?

"The only thing that holds you back from getting what you want is paying attention to what you don't want."
– Abraham-Hicks

I love Saturday Night Live (SNL). I'm sure you've heard of it. If you haven't, it's an awesome comedy show that comes on every Saturday. Talented comedians put on skits to live audiences every week.

One skit I'm fond of was done by actors Will Ferrell and Andy Samberg.

It's a musical skit called "Cool Guys Don't Look at Explosions."

Great title, right!

The main lyrics of the song go like this:

"Cool guys don't look at explosions, they blow things up, then walk away."

They sing these lyrics while showing famous actors like Denzel Washington, in well-known films, blowing things up, walking away, and never looking back at the explosion.

It's pretty ridiculous, but also makes them look very cool.

I try and remember this skit when I start to dwell on my past mistakes or any regrets.

It's not to say we shouldn't address our feelings or change our bad behavior, but do not let the past consume you, and prevent you from achieving the success you deserve.

Do not focus on where you have been, but where you want to go. Too many of us are living in the past. We look back at past mistakes, the words we forgot to say, or the person we should have been.

My friend, don't let the past keep you from future. Don't let the people that might have hurt you have that control over your life. Don't let a past mistake keep you from your destiny.

Just like the SNL skit, we may have blown some stuff up, but we need to turn around, walk away, and never look back.

Perhaps you are dealing with something this very moment that's holding you back. Some bad habit, or past mistake. Or perhaps a broken relationship.

No, we shouldn't ignore an issue or relationship, but do so right away. Don't wait another day to mend a relationship or confront a bad habit. Doing so will help us move on and away from our explosive past, and ensure we never look back.

Now, just imagine yourself six months or a year from today after beginning your own journey towards *Conquest*.

As you look back on the last six or twelve months, what do you want your life to look like? What have you accomplished? Who have you helped?

Have you left a legacy or written that book you've always wanted to write?

What goals or dreams have come true?

My hope is that you pick up this book six months or a year from now and ask yourself these questions with mind-blowing answers.

Because this book will have helped you self-reflect and discover.

It will have helped you find your inner passions and desires.

It will have helped you believe in yourself enough to set big, scary goals.

It will have helped you overcome your fear and doubt by taking massive action.

It will have helped you commit to your path and continue to learn and grow as an individual.

It will have helped you strengthen your health to unbelievable levels.

It will have helped you grow and unstoppable faith.

It will have helped you leave a lasting legacy.

It will have helped you remember all that you learn, so you can be your best self, every day.

Yes, this is my hope for you, my friend. That is why I've written this book.

If just one element of *Conquest* reaches your heart, I'll have done what I set out to do.

If just one person is touched by these words, I'll have done my job.

Life is a gift. Do not waste it. Use it to help others. You'll be able to help others the most by becoming your best self.

So, go and conquer your life with *Conquest* and leave a lasting legacy.

Thanks so much for reading

Wow, you finished the book. Thanks so much for taking the time to read *Conquest*. It means the world to me and I truly hope it has inspired you.

I am already working on my next book and plan to have many revisions of *Conquest* as well. To make these future edits the very best possible, I would love your input.

Would you please take just a few minutes to leave a helpful review of *Conquest* on Amazon?

Thanks so much!!!

-Aaron Gendle

Launch Team Crew

Thanks so much for helping make *Conquest* a success! I could not have done it without you …

Alex Lewis

Amber Lynn Bracken

Andy Gregory

Annie Sanger Bentley

Azzam Kamal

Belinda Gendle

Bhanu Nagpal

Brian Suttle

Brittany Sanger

Cheryl Gonseth

Christina Davis

Christine Martin

Danni Duff

Debbie Carroll BeLieu

Denette Stoll

Dianna Gray

Erin Virchow-Perrine

Hassan Bethea

Hayley Bruner

Holly McClintic

Holly Reneé

Jackie Azzara

Janice Burns

Janice Sanger

Jessi Cash

Jessie Coe

Jim Renke

Jill Martine

Joshua D. Girard

Kathe Easter- Fosnaugh

Katie Simmons

Kyle Sanger

Laura Phelps

Lisa Baum

LuAnne Longo

Lynn McGee

Mary Lou Killebrew

Megan A Johnson

Natalie Sanger Gendle

Nidhi Kadam

Nonie Jones Walsh McGraw

Paulina Montero

Peter Cruz

Ravneet Ghuman

Sahil Kala

Sarah Ruby Tassi

Sharon Carson

Stacey Baughman

Stacey Lynn Hale

Talitha Michael

Tammy Ryan

Terrance Christopher Maigi

Terri Schmidt

Theresa Fowler Foust

Tim Gendle

Toni Sanger

Tony Nguyen

Tracey Guerrero

Tricia Kerns

Valerie Bimbi

References

Crohn's disease - Symptoms and causes. (n.d.). Retrieved from http://www.mayoclinic.org/diseases-conditions/crohns-disease/symptoms-causes/syc-20353304

Sifferlin, A. (2017, August 15). 13% of Americans Take Antidepressants. Retrieved from http://time.com/4900248/antidepressants-depression-more-common/

Nationwide Trends. (2015, June). Retrieved from https://www.drugabuse.gov/publications/drugfacts/nationwide-trends

Suicide data. (n.d.). Retrieved from http://www.who.int/mental_health/prevention/suicide/suicideprevent/en/

Morrissey, M. (2016, September 14). The Power of Writing Down Your Goals and Dreams. Retrieved from https://www.huffingtonpost.com/marymorrissey/the-power-of-writing-down_b_12002348.html

Schawbel, D. (2016, October 11). Grant Cardone: Why Obsession Trumps Passion When It Comes To Success. Retrieved from https://www.forbes.com/sites/danschawbel/2016/10/11/grant-cardone-why-obsession-trumps-passion-when-it-comes-to-success/#3320d06b396e

18 Facts about Goals and their Achievement. (n.d.). Retrieved from http://www.goalband.co.uk/goal-achievement-facts.html

Peri, C. (n.d.). Sleep Loss: 10 Surprising Effects. Retrieved from https://www.webmd.com/sleep-disorders/features/10-results-sleep-loss

FastStats - Deaths and Mortality. (2017, May 22). Retrieved from https://www.cdc.gov/nchs/fastats/deaths.htm

Hyman, M. (2014, November 7). Why I am a Pegan – or Paleo-Vegan – and Why You Should Be Too! Retrieved from http://drhyman.com/blog/2014/11/07/pegan-paleo-vegan/

Horsley, K. (2016). Unlimited Memory: How to Use Advanced Learning Strategies to Learn Faster, Remember More and Be More Productive. TCK Publishing.

Cardone, G. (2011). The 10X Rule: The Only Difference Between Success and Failure (1 edition). Hoboken, N.J: Wiley.

Cardone, G. (2016). *Be Obsessed or Be Average*. New York: Portfolio.

Percentage of global drug users that have used either legal or illegal drugs within selected time periods as of 2017. (n.d.). Retrieved from https://www.statista.com/statistics/748184/global-drug-use-of-legal-and-illegal-drugs/

Zeratsky, K. (2014, November 7). Is juicing healthier than eating whole fruits or vegetables? Retrieved from https://www.mayoclinic.org/healthy-lifestyle/nutrition-and-healthy-eating/expert-answers/juicing/faq-20058020

Joel Osteen (2018, October 15) Retrieved from https://en.wikipedia.org/wiki/Joel_Osteen

Olsteen, J. (2016). The Power of I Am: Two Words That Will Change Your Life Today (1 edition). New York, N.Y: Faith Words.

N. (s.d.). Retrieved from https://www.brainyquote.com